ADAPTIVE MECHANISMS IN MIGRAINE: A COMPREHENSIVE SYNTHESIS IN EVOLUTION

BREAKING THE MIGRAINE CODE

ADAPTIVE MECHANISMS IN MIGRAINE: A COMPREHENSIVE SYNTHESIS IN EVOLUTION

BREAKING THE MIGRAINE CODE

Vinod Kumar Gupta

Physician, Gupta Medical Centre; S-407, Greater Kailash-II;
New Delhi, India

Nova Science Publishers, Inc.

New York

LIBRARY OF CONGRESS CATALOGING-IN-PUBLICATION DATA
Adaptive mechanisms in migraine / Vinod Kumar Gupta (editor).
  p. ; cm.
Includes index.
ISBN 978-1-60456-298-9 (softcover)
1. Migraine. I. Gupta, Vinod Kumar, 1972-
[DNLM: 1. Migraine Disorders--etiology. 2. Migraine Disorders--physiopathology. 3. Brain--physiology. WL 344 A221 2008]
RC392.A33 2008
616.8'4912--dc22

                                    2008019728

Published by Nova Science Publishers, Inc. ✛ *New York*

Dharam & Saran
Anjali & Vivek

CONTENTS

PREFACE

Errors may lurk even in our best tested theories. It is the responsibility of the professional to search for these errors. – Neil McIntyre, Karl Popper

Migraine has evolved into a giant puzzle and its research literature comprises a vast loosely-linked enterprise challenging human problem-solving capacity. Forty years ago, the exponentially rapid burgeoning of the scientific literature with only marginal practical utility was presaged.[1] As one of the commonest neurological / medical disorder, migraine certainly qualifies for this sober reflection. With some of the most colorful personalities in history having been afflicted with migraine, lay and the professional fascination for the disorder and its elusive mystery has never dimmed over the last two millennia. With dedicated teams of highly-qualified scientists in many countries studying the disorder in a systematic fashion over the last several decades and despite substantial resources having been spent to elucidate the disorder, at the beginning of the twenty-first century migraine research still remains primitive. The advent of advanced neuroimaging in the late twentieth century raised hopes of a quick resolution to what appeared to be a simple neurological problem. Such hopes based on technology -- that I label as the 'wow' factor, nevertheless, flattered only to deceive and finally proved unfounded and quite diversionary. The utility of the inexhaustible research literature of migraine has indeed become marginal. *The sheer breadth of treatments approved or suggested for migraine is in parallel with the starkly limited understanding of its genesis.* Empiricism and confusion reign in migraine therapeutics.

How does science approach that which is apparently undecipherable? With no clue to the basic physiological anomaly in migraine, researchers turned to nosology in order to give credibility to their research efforts. Migraine and other

---

[1] M. Burton. Science and Contemporary Society. University of Notre Dame Press, 1967.

primary vascular headaches stand out as a unique example among clinical entities in which an entirely subjective classification has been repeatedly heralded as a substantial and substantive advance. The International Headache Classification (2004) has placed the study of the pathophysiologic basis of migraine and other primary vascular headaches squarely on the back-burner. By legitimizing clinical and laboratory including genetic research directed to the many *so-called* variants of migraine or idiopathic vascular headache as distinct clinical entities, the International Headache Classification has almost ensured that a comprehensive theory might never emerge. While tension headache has "advanced" to tension-type headache and then to chronic tension-type headache (CTTH) or chronic daily headache (CDH), we remain as ignorant of the 'entity' as ever before; that CTTH or CDH differs fundamentally from migraine is one of the major well-entrenched myths in this field. *New words or terms do not automatically enhance knowledge or understanding*.

The headache and the other accompaniments of migraine are remarkably protean in nature. The severity and duration of pain during different migraine attacks commonly differ even in the same patient. The methodology of the randomized controlled trial (RCT) assumes that the parameter (more correctly, variable) under evaluation would remain steady over the period of observation. *By encouraging RCT in primary vascular headaches, the non-suitability of migraine to the methodology of the RCT has been obscured to a non-issue.* Randomization is not a scientific method but an invaluable strategy for mathematically managing uncertainty. The mathematical basis of the RCT through statistics and its inability to distinguish between relatively small effects has generated a very large mass of data in primary headache research that is not only often conflicting but also misguiding. Migraine remains a classic example of a clinical entity that has not yielded its secrets to statistical legerdemain. *Perhaps in no other clinical entity has the immeasureable proven so much more important than the measureable.*[2]

There is no central idea in current migraine research to elaborate a general theory which, in turn, could ultimately lead to creation of a unifying hypothesis that collects the various strands of evidences into a coherent and logically defensible intelligible synthesis. Current pathogenetic concepts of migraine, in particular *cortical spreading depression* (CSD), do not focus on the precise onset of the attack. Neither the aura nor the headache represents the true beginning of a migraine attack. The primary or causal physiological alteration underlying

---

[2] The recipe for perpetual ignorance is to be satisfied with your opinions and content with your knowledge. – Elbert Hubbard.

migraine lies in the 'pre-prodromal' phase, the variable interim between exposure to the headache-provoking stimulus or situation and the onset of the migraine prodrome. The migraine prodrome itself can last several hours to a few days. *Since CSD is believed to underlie both the migrainous scintillating scotoma as well as the headache, it cannot be regarded as an early or initial 'pre-prodromal' physiological event.* A generalized and particularly cardiac autonomic dysfunction has been established in migraine patients; we have absolutely no clue how to link this autonomic feature (or pupillary anomalies) to CSD. In this manner, several large unbridgeable gaps exist in the chain of scientific logic in current migraine research.

The biology of migraine is not the study of laboratory 'markers' but the elucidation of physiological forces (trait and/or state factors) that push (precipitate) or pull (predispose) patients towards aura/headache state or aura/headache-free state.[3] Study of pathophysiology of migraine has been hitherto confined to analyses of diverse attack precipitating and remitting factors and uncertain postulations about recorded laboratory aberrations into presumptive causal algorithms. *The key cranial physiological system involved in migraine remains unidentified.* Migraine attacks occur during stress and, more commonly, after cessation of stress. I have earlier proposed that a physiological neuroendocrine 'system' comprised of well-regulated parallel activation of the vasopressinergic, intrinsic brain serotonergic, and intrinsic brain noradrenergic systems constitutes an important adaptive mechanism that governs vascular integrity, antinociception, behavior and overall function during stressful occasions, including migraine attacks. Such a conceptual template can be used to segregate the vast phenomenology of migraine into primary pathogenetic or secondary non-pathogenetic divisions; non-pathogenetic migrainous phenomena can be further subdivided into adaptive or concomitant (epiphenomenal / bystander) physiological events. Nausea and/or vomiting, facial pallor, Raynaud's phenomenon, episodic daytime sleepiness, and relative hypotension (both spontaneous as well as induced by prophylactic anti-migraine pharmacologic agents) likely reflect the non-pathogenetic (adaptive or epiphenomenal) clinical components of migraine. Since nausea/vomiting commonly aborts migraine attacks – with or without aura -- the pathophysiological basis and the biological purpose of aura/headache and nausea/vomiting of migraine is very unlikely to be identical. Further, exogenous magnesium does not readily cross the intact blood-brain barrier (BBB) and decreases the permeability of the BBB. Magnesium

---

[3] Everything that can be counted does not necessarily count; everything that counts cannot necessarily be counted. – Albert Einstein.

depletion appears to serve an important cardiovascular adaptive function; its utility in migraine management is not convincing. Magnesium depletion, platelet activation, peripheral alterations in serotonin and catecholamine metabolism, hyper-responsiveness of brain noradrenergic, serotonergic, vasopressinergic, and dopaminergic systems, parasympathetic nevous system activation, pupillary miosis, and cutaneous allodynia probably represent some of the secondary adaptive physiological mechanisms operative in migraine.

A critical or central role for brain neuronal involvement in migraine pathogenesis appears unikely as established migraine preventive agents like atenolol, nadolol, and (to an extent) verapamil and aura-aborting agents such as nitroglycerine, nifedipine, and isoproterenol do not readily cross the intact BBB or significantly influence brain neuronal function. Antidepressants, including amitriptyline, induce brain noradrenergic and serotonergic hyperfunction, rendering highly unlikely that such brain states underlie migraine. Migraine preventive agents modulate the primary physiological aberration. In contrast to migraine abortive agents (in particular, triptans) whose site of action remains uncertain on the 'efferent limb' of migraine, the site of action of some migraine preventive agents unambiguously appears to lie outside the brain on the 'afferent limb'.

Elucidation of adaptive physiological mechanisms in migraine can rationalize its important epidemiological, clinical, and pharmacological features, and, sow the seeds for evolution of an integrative synthesis that, in turn, might herald the creation of a comprehensive thought framework and research vision for migraine. *Such efforts can be easily dismissed as improper science or mere speculations without proper scientific background / backing or data. That science is merely data is a truly stunting vision of a grand intellectual enterprise. Data only reflect the terminal results of cogitation, observation, and experimentation. With the overwhelming of medical research by mathematical statistics, data are no longer steeped in biological importance.[4] Data do not precede or supplant a careful reflection about the problem. Currently, we gather data and then set about trying to make sense of our results. Logic, necessarily, goes out of the window. The science of migraine currently requires much more reflection, reflection free from the shackles of statistics, and, this book is no more than a tottering step in that direction.* To uncritically embrace mythical concepts – howsoever wrapped in statistics -- and to carry on thus indefinitely does not appear to be the right approach.

To grapple with migraine mechanisms is formidable, ambitious, almost arrogant impulse. Institutional support involving large self-organizing groups and tangible factors such as funding and laboratory space have not yet unlocked the migraine code. Natural laws become apparent only when science becomes abstract, bordering on art. While far from being a comprehensive tome on the subject, this book may best be regarded as an act of contemplative and inventive deconstruction – a form of insurrection[5] -- and a prelude to the final unravelling of one of the most enduring mysteries of Nature. The author has undertaken this almost impossible mission simply because someone had to undo the Gordian knot of migraine existing for -- and getting more complicated -- over two millennia.

I dedicate this book to the memory of my father, Dharam Prakash Gupta (1926-1981), former Professor & Head of Departments of Pathology & Bacteriology at Medical Colleges & Attached Group of Hospitals in Rajasthan (India) at Jaipur, Bikaner, Jodhpur, and Ajmer. He also worked as a research associate and taught at the Mallory Institute of Pathology, Boston, Massachusetts, U.S.A. (1963-1964). My mother, Saran, continues to be a source of inspiration and support for my dabblings in science and art. Migraine has consumed my mind and my life leaving me with lesser time than I would otherwise have devoted to my family and to my other whims. My wife, Anjali, currently Pathologist at Dubai Police Headquarters Force, Dubai, U.A.E., shares with me the dream of the unvieling of the ultimate truth about migraine. Anjali and my son, Vivek, have somehow managed to overlook the huge chunks of time that this effort has cost me and hopefully will forgive my inadequacies as a husband and as a father.

This preface woud be incomplete without a special word for the migraine patients who reposed great faith in my self-styled therapeutic abilities. "Where is your laboratory?" -- I have often been asked this question by some patients and many incredulous medical professionals. I do not, perhaps mercifully, have a research laboratory to justify the 'tag' of being labeled even as an amateur researcher. My 'laboratory' is the migraine patients themselves. Listening carefully to my migraine patients while incessantly analyzing the published literature set into process the mysterious wheels of cogitation, the identification of rhetoric, the weeding out of the dross, and the frantic clutching at the elusive slippery essence of migraine itself without any pre-conceived notion about its nature. Had I devoted the bulk of my energies towards the laboratory investigation

---

[4] Doctors should not engage in an "intellectual lobotomy that equates statistical significance with biological, physiological, or quantitative importance. – A.R. Feinstein,. Hypertension, 1985;7:313- 318.

[5] Insurrection is an art, and like all arts it has its laws. – L. Trotsky.

of migraine I would have long since been lost in the bewitching woods of migraine-related data. This overview could then not have possibly been conceived.

Some of the best intellects in history have challenged the ostensibly impregnable fortress of migraine, leaving their impressions as templates for the future. "The most valuable lesson knowledge that can teach us is that its creation depends upon a line of human relationships and traditions that go far back in to the past. That continuity is an unbroken thread. It links cultures and peoples; it brings tolerance and understanding; it delivers hope and compassion" – Anonymous. The templates of the past formed essential stepping stones in my quixotic quest for the basis of migraine.[6] *Science in medicine, however, carries hidden in its folds an intolerance, an irreverence, an impatience, a sledgehammer-like either/or approach through technology and RCT-related statistical mathematics that is often ill-suited to approach the unknown*. My failure as a physician to further specialize into any one of the several branches of Internal Medicine is probably the most critical investigator-related variable in the endeavor to understand migraine. Confined to a minute part of the body, the knowledge of specialists of the rest of the body is so rudimentary that they become incapable of thoroughly understanding even that fragment in which they specialize -- *Alexis Carrell*. Understanding migraine requires both consummate depth and breadth of knowledge in medicine.

Finally, if I may allow myself the privilege to address the unborn generations of future researchers, another trait required for deviant or 'Copernican' thinking is the refusal to attend Medical Conferences. Medicine is a social science and medical conferencing is the art of ensuring that nobody gets ahead of the pack. As grand social events, medical conferences bristle with ideas of human identity and entity involving fantasy, manipulation, subtle construction of dogma and stealthy invention of myths. Defeaning applauses and standing ovations mean everyone (or nearly everyone) is in synchrony. Science, however, is not democratic. True progress in science, however, requires the daring to view phenomenology differently, to give birth to and to maintain a disquieting dys-synchrony, to confront and not to be overawed by convention or history or authority, and to remain curious and imaginative. In medicine, an additional requisite is the ability to distance oneself from mathematics and to place statistical significance at a much lower rung than its presently hallowed status. In the simplistic quest for symmetry and patterns in

Nature, mathematics reigns supreme. Much of medical research in the last several decades has been mathematical rather than clinical. Whatever is statistically significant is certainly publishable; equally certainly, it is not biologically or medically original. Like pun in words, mathematical patterns are pun in numbers. Neither pun in words nor pun in numbers can ever be original in medicine.

This synthesis is the direct outcome of the publication and dissemination of my project on migraine by the Rolex Awards Committee, 1990, Switzerland. The framework for the synthesis was conceived between 1975- 1989 and continues to be refined. If not for the presentation for the Rolex Awards project in 1989, the present work may never have surfaced. While this synthesis might seem a personal dream come true, the implications for science and humankind are far more important.

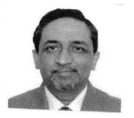

Great sums of money are wasted every year on scientific research in America as well as in Europe...Neither laboratories, nor apparatus, nor organization can give to scientists the surroundings indispensable to their success...We have an almost irresistible tendency to select the subjects of our investigations for their technical facility and clearness rather than for their importance...A work of art has never been produced by a committee of artists, nor a great discovery made by a committee of scholars. The syntheses needed for the progress of our knowledge of man should be elaborated in a single brain.
Alexis Carrel (1873-1944). Man, The Unknown. Hamish Hamilton, Ltd., London,
1959.

----

6 The reasonable man adapts himself to the world; the unreasonable one persists in trying to adapt the world to himself. Therefore, all progress depends on the unreasonable man. G.B. Shaw (Man and Superman).

ABBREVIATIONS

ACTH   adrenocorticotropic hormone
ASD   atrial septal defect
ANS   autonomic nervous system
AVP   arginine vasopressin
BBB   blood-brain barrier
CDH   chronic daily headache
CNS   central nervous system
CGRP   calcitonin-gene related peptide
CSF   cerebrospinal fluid
CNV   contingent negative variation
CSD   cortical spreading depression
CTTH   chronic tension type headache
CVS   cyclic vomiting syndrome
EEG   electrocencephalography(ic)
GON   greater occipital nerve
5-HT   5-hydroxytryptamine
IOP   intraocular pressure
ICA   internal carotid artery
MA+   migraine with aura
MA-   migraine without aura
MRI   magnetic resonance imaging
$Mg+^2$ magnesium (ionic)
m-CPP m-chlorophenylpiperazine
NO   nitric oxide
NE   norepinephrine
OM   ophthalmoplegic migraine

V 1   ophthalmic division of trigeminal nerve
PNS   parasympathetic nervous system
PFO   patent foramen ovale
POAG   primary open angle glaucoma
RCT   randomized controlled trial
REM   rapid eye movement
RSD   retinal spreading depression
SNS   sympathetic nervous system
SSRI   selective serotonin reuptake inhibitors
TxA_2 thromboxane A_2

Chapter 1

BACKGROUND: WHAT AILS MIGRAINE RESEARCH?

The pathogenesis of migraine remains uncertain and, currently, its therapy is completely empirical [1]. Whether migraine is a specific disorder (clinical entity) or a non-specific response to a variety of responses is also undecided. Consequently, efforts to prevent migraine vary widely and might involve pharmacological agents [2] or scalp injection of botulinum toxin [3] or closure of patent foramen ovale (PFO) or atrial septal defect (ASD) [4] or greater occipital nerve (GON) injection [5] or GON stimulation. Medication abuse is frequent seen in migraine patients; triptans and opiates are commonly involved [6]. Central brain or thalamic or brain stem neuronal dysfunction possibly related to cortical spreading depression (CSD) or involvement of the midbrain periaqueductal gray is currently believed to underlie both the aura as well as the headache in migraine patients [1,7-11]. The occipital cortex is generally *believed* to generate the visual symptoms of migraine aura, including paradoxically *both* uniocular as well as binocular (*presumedly*, homonymously distributed) scintillating scotomata [12]. Although research thinking has swung from the vascular to the neurologic or the neurogenic theories, a key acknowledged limitation of neurologic / neurogenic theories for migraine is the signficantly delayed development of migraine aura or headache in a variety of clinical circumstances and situations, including stress [13,14].

A large body of evidence *appears* to support the role of brain CSD as a key component of the migraine pathogenetic cascade [8,9,12,15-18]. The central postulate in the CSD-related pathogenetic algorithm for migraine is the presumed role of intrinsic or brain noradrenergic activation [17,18]. Although the biobehavioral model of migraine involving CSD [17,18] has underpinned much research effort for the last two decades, important clinical, experimental, and pharmacological features challenge this research premise [19-22]. *The available migraine research literature does not answer an important question related to its pathogenesis. The most plausible link of CSD is with the aura / headache phase of migraine. CSD has not been postulated to occur in the pre-prodromal stage or the prodromal stage of migraine. What physiological aberration, then, underlies the pre-prodromal and the prodromal phases of migraine, and, why should such aberration develop in the first instance? Does this early aberration have any link to CSD? Also, since nausea and/or vomiting is a cardinal feature of migraine, it would be invaluable to know how CSD could possibly stimulate the vomiting centre in the medulla. Regrettably, all we have currently is hazy ideas about these aspects of CSD and migraine pathophysiology. A generation of neuroscientists devoted to primary headache research has accepted CSD as the basis of migraine, but this acceptance is purely notional or speculative, not even circumstantial. Nevertheless, CSD has permeated and dominated ("enraptured") the psyche of most primary headache researchers and captured their imagination, making them both unwilling as well as incapable of entertaining any alternative explanation.*

Recently, closure of PFO/ASD has resulted in precipitation of frequent/daily migraine with aura headaches in some patients; such cardiac intervention apparently has nothing to do with CSD. The link between PFO closure and prevention of recurrent strokes in cryptogenic stroke or migraine attacks is too nebulous to stand critical scrutiny. The case for an adaptive function for PFO itself is being gradually built.

*Although homonymous scintillating scotomata have **never** been unequivocally described in migraine patients, for most migraine researchers, it is currently inconceivable that the migrainous scintillating scotomata might not originate at the occipital cortex. **At this point, most migraine researchers have confused the distribution of the negative homonymous hemianopia with that of the positive scintillating scotoma, and, have made a most unfortunate conceptual error with such neuro-ophthalmological substitution/assumption.*** Since lay patients do not understand the anatomical basis of uniocular or binocular vision, the revelation regarding distribution of migrainous scintillating scotoma must necessarily come from either a migraine patient with sufficient medical background or by asking patients so afflicted to confirm uniocular/binocular distribution of the positive scotoma by covering both eyes in turn. *This simple measure has not been detailed to date, the reason for which is the absolute belief of the migraine research community about the origin of the scintillating scotoma. **Another critical issue is the dismaying neglect of the importance of the blood-brain barrier (BBB) in*** *migraine pharmacotheraqpy and pathophysiology. One of the most carefully nurtured secret of migarine research is that atenolol is as effective as propranolol in prevention of migraine attacks; since atenolol does not freely cross the BBB or significantly alter brain neuronal function, this feature strikes at the heart of brain-centric theories of migraine.* Myths[1] and assumptions abound in in migraine research, as in most other human endeavors, serving an important intellectual function, i.e., to fill the gaps between our expectations, our uncertainties, and the ground reality or the truth; paradoxically, this bridging of our ignorances comforts but impedes true progress.

In the subsequent chapters, I will endeavor to signpost those aspects of migraine that *must* be rationalized in order to develop a comprehensive and overarching theory for migraine [19][22] and will also present a preliminary framework for evolution of the concept of adaptive / protective physiological processes operating in migraine.

The contemplation of things as they are, without error or confusion, without substitution or imposture, is in itself a nobler thing than a whole harvest of inventions. -- Sir Francis Bacon.

---

[1] The principal psychosocial function of myths is to offer a vicarious resolution of the ignorance that lies between our insecurities and our expectations. – Claude Lévi-Strauss

Chapter 2

QUEST FOR A NEW RESEARCH PARADIGM FOR MIGRAINE: 'WHY' AND 'HOW'

The need for a broad concept of migraine, not related to the vascular or neurological (brain) systems has been clearly elucidated [13,23]. Fresh, out-of-the-box or lateral thinking unlinked to existing theoretical concepts is essential for any meaningful progress in migraine pathophysiology as well as for the rationalization of the massive extant data bank.

The phenomenology of primary vascular headaches including migraine has been extensively described in the field as well as in the laboratory. The symptomatology of migraine forms the uncertain basis of the elaborate and seemingly sophisticated nosologic system – both the current [24] and the previous versions. *To maintain that a distinct pathophysiologic mechanism will ultimately be discovered for each of the nosologic entities currently delineated by the new version of the classification of the International Headache Society [24] appears to be nothing but a form of irrational scepticism [22].* A phenomenological (symptoms-based) classification of primary headaches cannot be equated with a comprehensive pathophysiological 'system'. Although identification of narrow homogeneous groups or clinical phenotypes and development of a comprehensive pathophysiologic system may be closely linked, these two approaches might also work at cross-purposes.[1] *Such kind of 'splitting' of clinical 'entities' renders the creation of a unifying hypothesis for primary vascular headaches practically impossible. To maintain that migraine with aura (MA+) and migraine without aura (MA-) are distinct nosologic entities with*

---

[1] H.M. van Pragg, M.H. Lader, O.J. Rafaelsen, E.J. Sachar (editors). Handbook of Biological Psychiatry. Part I. Marcel Dekker, Inc. New York, 1981.

significant pathophysiological differences while most migraine patients experience both variants and respond to similar therapies is yet another form of irrationality. Migraine patients only rarely do not have tension-type headaches at other periods of their lives. Drawing an analogy from cardiovascular medicine, the atheromatous plaque underlies all clinical expressions of coronary heart disease including the two anginal variants, effort induced angina and angina at rest; there is no claim that the aginal variants are distinct clinical entities. *Contemporary migraine research stands where cardiovascular medicine once stood before the discovery of the atheromatous plaque* [22].

Triptans, besides CSD, have also seized the imagination of most migraine researchers. From being only abortive medications for long, migraine research has recently flirted with the preventive value of triptans. Triptans are currently believed to work at multiple targets, *within* the brain and at both *central* and *peripheral* terminals of trigeminal "pain-sensory" fibres. Admittedly, the study of 5-HT receptor subtypes has advanced tremendously along with use of triptans in migraine. For several decades, it was assumed that the migraine-aborting action of triptans was specific/selective to migraine; indeed, the importance of triptans to migraine pathophysiology rose in parallel with this belief. Challenging this concept and bringing the enthusiasts back to base is the recent observation that triptans can attenuate non-cranial/trigeminal somatic as well as visceral pain in behavioral (but not acute nocieptive) models of persistent inflammatory pain.[2] Thus begins the disconcerting process of reorientation of widely held migraine-centric concepts about triptans and their role in pain that overrode and limited our thinking for long. *The pharmaceutical industry has a deep fiscal interest in the triptan bandwagon and a skewed view of scientific progress – the bottom-line is always far more important.† Any progress that does not shore up profits is inconsequential as far as the industry is concerned. Industry sponshorsip of published papers and medical careers is a pernicious and disquieting influence that insidiously shapes the minds of the targeted community – the prescribers. Triptans have been propelled to the forefront in migraine therapeutics as well as research largely through the overt and covert support of the industry.*

Further elucidation of 'what' of migraine carries the subtle but unfortunate paradox that additional data will contribute little to our comprehension of the disorder unless extant data is arranged into a vast intelligible synthesis ('why' and 'how') that places key elements of the entity in a logically-defensible, perspective-enhancing, and hopefully insight- and experiment-generating bio-

---

[2] A.H. Ahn & A.I. Basbaum. J Neurosci 2006;26:8332-8; T. Nikai, A.I. Basbaum, A.H. Ahn. Pain 2008;139:533-40.

compatible model. Such conceptual groundwork is an important part of the migraine research process that cannot be supplanted by randomized controlled clinical trials (RCT) or by meta-analysis of RCTs [19-22,25-28]. Also, refining the accounts of the headache of migraine patients – exploding vs. imploding headache[3] – neither really offers any fresh insight into migraine mechanisms nor resolves the apparently insoluble intracranial vs. extracranial innervation involvement debate. *The lure of novel words notwithstanding, scientific advance and sensibility generally has nothing to do with linguistic finesse.*

As Claude Bernard and Peter Medawar have emphasized, every systematic inquiry must start with a preconceived idea and a careful phrasing of the research question [29,30]. Although stress is the most commonly cited cause of migraine [13,31], as in other areas of medicine, generally, the word 'stress' carries little or no utility, serving mainly as a euphemism for ignorance – a confusing pseudo-explanation confounding rational thought [32]. In migraine pathophysiology, the term 'stress' has been used, perhaps reflexly or unthinkingly, as a substitutive pseudo-biological term that has undermined the significances of both post-stress aura and headache as well as the typical neuro-anatomic lateralization (unilateral, bilateral, or side-shift) of headache [33]. Nevertheless, "Good medicine is indivisible, has always been holistic in the sense that it considered the whole patient, has always seen the patient balanced between opposing forces pushing him towards health or disease the ability to continue to function in the period immediately after acute injury.and the variations in the effects of the same injury in the same individual from time to time just as between individuals is unlikely to be unifactorial or a 'hopelessly complex' obfuscation, but is probably the result of a meticulously orchestrated parallel activation of multiple physiological (secondary stress or adaptive) processes" [34]. As related to migraine, 'stress' is not a hopelessly complex obfuscation; on the other hand, stress-related physiological aberrations hold the key to understanding migraine. Furthermore, the term 'biological' is not synonymous with 'physiological,' 'organic,' or 'nonenvironmental,' as has often seemed the case in the medical literature [35]. While the biology of migraine is at its infancy, migraine researchers lay great (but misplaced) emphasis on the discovery of a 'biological marker' for the entity in the laboratory. A series of laboratory measurements, labeled rather prematurely as 'biological markers', have intermittently held attention of migraine researchers for varying intervals: neurochemicals, neuropeptides, platelets, evoked potentials, pupillary aberrations, neuroimaging features, and genetic linkages. Laboratory

---

[3] M. Jakubowski et al. Pain 2006;125:286-295.

medicine is essentially 'reductionist', the exclusive focus on one or two factors generally leading to neglect of the whole [13,36,37].

The biology of an illness is the elucidation of the forces that push an individual towards the disease or the disease-free state. The first step in the evolution of a biologically-relevant overarching theory for migraine is the elucidation of the physiological forces (processes) that push or pull the patient towards the aura/headache or the aura/headache-free state, significantly delay onset of the migraine attack (with or without aura) for several hours or a few days after exposure to diverse attack-provoking stimuli, allow patients to function despite the attack-related morbidity, keep patients in extended (but variable) remissions, and prevent attacks in four-fifths of the general population.[36] Up till now, all documented physiological perturbations of migraine have been rather simplistically consigned to the general cause/effect template thereby blurring the distinction between the two. In the absence of a distinction between primary and secondary physiological events, it has also remained impossible to categorize secondary physiological events or 'effects' into useful (adaptive) or concomitant ('innocent bystander' or epiphenomenon) categories.

In summary, a neuroendocrine adaptive 'system' has been suggested to maintain vascular integrity, antinociception, and behavior during migraine attack-related vasodilatory antidromic trigeminal nerve discharge, the proposed components of which include sympathetic hyperfunction coupled to enhanced bioavailability of arginine-vasopressin (AVP) and serotonin (5-HT), with the onset of headache representing overwhelming ('fatigue') of the 'system' [36,37]. The physiological system(s) primarily affected in migraine must be, therefore, afforded a considerable (but limited and eventually exhaustible) degree of protection by homeostatic defense mechanisms, thereby allowing the subject to continue to function despite the stressful stimulus or situation; this protection is obviously unlimited or inexhaustible in the majority of the general population who are not susceptible to migraine. *The conceptual divide between pathogenetic and adaptive or 'protective' physiologic mechanisms in migraine has the potential to enhance our understanding of its pathophysiological basis.* Such thinking involves a profound shift in focus -- regarding the mechanistic basis -- from the aura/headache state to the aura/headache-free state.

If facts deviate, they must be forced to conform; if the facts prove recalcitrant, they can be imagined away since only the theory is true. Perhaps some day the facts will prove inescapable – W.A. Glaser (Lancet 341;805-812, 1993).

Chapter 3

NAUSEA/VOMITING-VASOPRESSIN NEXUS IN MIGRAINE

Science may be described as the art of systematic over-simplification.

Karl Popper.

Nausea and/or vomiting are cardinal and diagnostic features of migraine attacks, both with and without aura; other forms of primary headaches are generally not associated with nausea and/or vomiting [24]. In migraine with aura (MA+), headache, nausea and/or vomiting, and photophobia generally follow neurological aura symptoms either directly or within an hour [24]. The mechanism of origin of migrainous nausea and/or vomiting remains unknown. Also, the biological role or purpose of nausea and/or vomiting in migraine is uncertain.

Conventionally, early nausea and/or vomiting in migraine attacks is assumed to reflect an outcome of activation of the same putative pathogenetic cascade in migraine as is the neurologic aura or the headache, with spreading depression-related orbitofrontal cortical, hypothalamic, and brain stem activation along with 5-HT release forming the final common pathway [17,18,38]. Hypothalamic stimulation and neuroendrocrine alterations including AVP release during migraine attacks are believed to be consistent with Leão's concept of spreading electric depression [39]. In practical terms, current understanding of migraine pathophysiology assumes that spreading depression -- *believed* to be initiated at onset of migraine attacks at the brain cortex -- spreads to the brain stem and induces nausea and/or vomiting. Drummond and Granston further believe that nausea and headache, two key symptoms of migraine, interact pathogenetically by reinforcing each other in a vicious circle during attacks [40]. The cyclic vomiting syndrome (CVS) also is believed to have the same pathophysiological basis as migraine [41, 42]. Besides, gastric stasis has been suggested to underlie nausea of migraine; however, gastric stasis is more pronounced between migraine attacks than during attacks [43]. Additionally, triptans relieve attack-related nausea but worsen gastric stasis [43]. Next, diabetic autonomic neuropathy is commonly associated with gastroparesis but the diabetic state appears unlinked to migraine. Conversely, hypoglycemia (rather than hyperglycemia) is a well-known precipitating factor for migraine attacks [13]. Although, there is general agreement that nausea and/or vomiting of migraine is central in origin, no conceptual or functional / teleologic distinction has been hitherto drawn in the analysis of migraine pathophysiology between the biological bases of headache and that of nausea and/or vomiting.

Over 2000 years ago, Hippocrates described "...vomiting, when it became possible, was able to divert the pain and render it more moderate" [44]. In 1790, Tissot wrote: "... vomiting might herald the termination of the headache" [45]. There is general consensus that vomiting during migraine, particularly in children, is often associated with subjective improvement or complete termination of the attack [46,47]. *The mechanistic basis of amelioration or termination of migraine headache attacks by nausea and/or vomiting is currently unknown.*

Emesis clearly has an antidiuretic action indicating increased AVP release [48, 49]. Nausea itself -- even without vomiting -- is accompanied by intense and rapid AVP release, as is also stress or pain [48-50]. Virtually instantaneous increases in plasma AVP from 100 to 1000 times basal level are not unusual even when the nausea is transient and unaccompanied by vomiting or changes in blood pressure. Mild nausea can distort physiological AVP responses because nausea is a more potent and predominating stimulus to AVP release [48-50]. Nausea-mediated AVP release dominates over concomitant inhibition by water loading (osmolar) or ethanol (pharmacologic); specificity of nausea-mediated AVP release is indicated by absence of significant increases in plasma AVP -- in contrast to human subjects -- in rats (which lack an emetic reflex) given relatively large doses of apomorphine [50]. As part of the adaptive system that can delay the onset of or abort migraine attacks, AVP likely promotes vasomotor control, antinociception, and behavior control [37]. As reviewed, the antinociceptive effect of AVP is experimentally well-defined, clinically useful, and involves interaction with endogenous opiates [37]. Nausea and/or vomiting probably represent an important anticipatory or attack-related neuroendocrinological mechanism designed to delay onset of and to limit impact of aura/headache attacks in migraine patients [37, 51, 52].

Pallor of the skin is a frequent accompaniment of autonomic activation during nausea and/or vomiting and is commonly noted during migraine attacks [46, 53]. Elevations of plasma AVP sufficient to cause facial pallor have been shown in migraine attacks [54]. Diuretics or fluid loading do not affect occurrence of menstrual migraine attacks; the theoretical basis for regarding skin pallor (and attack-related fluid retention or platelet aggregation) as a physiological trade-off has been discussed [37,55]. Renal and extra-renal manifestations in migraine patients probably represent concomitant side effects of an adaptive physiological change. Fine-tuning of the mutually opposing influences of AVP and cortisol secretion on sodium and water balance at the renal tubule (possibly modulated additionally by endogenous opioid peptides, exercise, estrogens, nicotine, dopamine, and atrial natriuretic peptide affecting either release of AVP and or the renal tubular system) may allow appropriate fluid homeostasis in the majority of patients with spontaneous migraine, while exerting additive adaptive influences at other sites, including the cranial vessels. While the 'vascular hypothesis' has fallen into disfavor largely because many migraine patients manifest pallor rather than the expected flushing (a reflection of extracranial vasodilatation) during attacks, facial circulatory changes and thermographic aberrations at any point of time simply reflect the balance between systemic and regional vasoconstrictive and vasodilatory influences. Facial pallor or flushing during migraine -- like the headache or the aura (discussed further in this article) -- do not indicate the beginning of the attack but represent the end-result of a series of closely-regulated physiological influences. Additionally, AVP secretion is associated with increased bioavailablity of oxytocin [49]. A role for oxytocin in antinociception has only recently been appreciated [56,57].

AVP appears to be a key modulator of migraine; several facets of migraine phenomenology seem linked to stimulated or inhibited secretion of AVP [37] (Table 1): (i) Sleep has a complex influence upon migraine attacks. Sleep has a well-defined therapeutic effect on migraine headache [58-60]. Sleep commonly terminates migraine attacks; 14 out of 50 migraine patients could shorten their attacks by unscheduled daytime sleeping for ~2.5 hours [58]. In another study, 85% of migraineurs indicated that they chose to sleep or rest because of headache and 75% were forced to sleep or rest because of headache [60]. Sleep stimulates AVP secretion without any relation to electroencephalographic (EEG) sleep stage; significantly, such physiological elevation occurs at a time when redistribution of blood volume from the extremities to the central vessels would otherwise suppress AVP secretion [49]. Conversely, sleep can precipitate migraine. Migraine headache early in the morning or after brief periods of diurnal sleep [59,61] suggests a pathogenetic role for exhaustion or depletion of noradrenergic and/or

AVP systems [62]. Rapid eye movement (REM) sleep is associated with autonomic nervous system (ANS) activation. The link between early morning migraine attacks and increased REM sleep [63] may lie in exhaustion/depletion of ANS as well as vasopressinergic systems in these predisposed patients. (ii) Amitriptyline, a fairly established migraine prophylactic agent in the 'proven' or 'well-accepted' category [2] (the evidence pre-dating the RCT-era), has a rapid prophylactic action in migraine that appears unrelated to the relatively delayed clinical alleviation of depression [64]. Migraine-preventive action of amitriptyline is uncertainly attributed to sedative, anti-depressant, anti-serotonergic, or calcium-channel blockade actions [65]. Tricyclic antidepressants, nevertheless, increase AVP release from the neurohypophysis [49] and also suppress REM sleep and increase REM sleep onset latency in depressed patients [63,66] (discussed further in this chapter). (iii) Some migraine patients improve with exercise [67,68]. Physical exercise increases plasma AVP levels [49]. (iv) Migraine patients may seek relief by smoking [69] while severe migraine headaches can develop after sudden discontinuation of nicotine gum [70]. Some people smoke to reduce dysphoria and anxiety [71]. Nicotine readily crosses the blood-brain barrier (BBB) and promotes release of AVP, β-endorphin, acetylcholine, norepinephrine (NE), dopamine, 5-HT, and adrenocorticotropic hormone (ACTH) [71]. Evidence for a potent antinociceptive effect of nicotine [72] is increasing and the rationale for using nicotine agonists as analgesics [73] is evolving.[1] The antinociceptive effect of nicotine appears to be mediated via nicotinic and mu-opioid receptors [72,73]. AVP likely subserves the neuroendocrine link between these two receptor systems [37]. (v) Migraine attacks (MA+ or MA-) that begin during pregnancy usually subside within three months [74,75] and a substantial fraction of female migraine patients progressively improves during pregnancy [76]. The fluid overload and relative hyponatremia of later stages of pregnancy [77] might restore or enhance AVP efficacy [78] and ameliorate migraine [37]. (vi) Frequency of migraine attacks generally decreases with increasing age [13,46,79], a feature that might be linked to progressive increase in plasma AVP concentration -- and incidence of hyponatremia -- with advancing years [37]. Paradoxically, acute hypoglycaemia, that frequently precipitates migraine attacks, is associated with non-osmotic AVP release.

Several well-known precipitants of migraine decrease AVP secretion, bioavailability, or efficacy [37] (table 1): (i) Fear or anxiety-related acute emotional stress may actively suppress AVP secretion [80,81] thereby setting the

---

[1] A patient with refractory migraine / CTTH with a short-term good response to nicotine gum has been recently described. [V.K. Gupta. Journal of Emergency Medicine 2007; 14(4):243-244.]

stage for both occurrence of migraine *during* stress [82] as well as the association between anxiety state (either alone or linked with depression) and migraine [83].

In contrast to acute experimental or real-life anxiety, prolonged or chronic anxiety state is invariably associated with ANS activation – clinically overt or covert. Phasic neuroendocrine – autonomic or vasopressinergic or both – depletion/exhaustion may predispose such patients to migraine attacks. (ii) Alcohol, a well-known precipitant of migraine [82], inhibits neurohypophyseal function. In rats chronically treated with ethanol, the level of AVP mRNA in the hypothalamis was markedly reduced and was unaffected by salt-loading [84]. (iii) Reserpine administered intramuscularly consistently causes profound release of 5-HT from platelets and precipitates migraine-like headaches in migraine patients [85,86]. Reserpine diminished the loss of AVP from the pituitary and the rise in urinary excretion of AVP that results from water deprivation [87]. (iv) Forty percent of migraine patients do not improve with pregnancy; of this subset, about two-thirds are unchanged and one-third worsen [88,89]. Placental vasopressinase degrades AVP; vasopressinase greatly increases during later stages of pregnancy, thereby reducing the bioavailability of AVP [90]. Also, women with migraine are more likely to have excessive nausea and vomiting during pregnancy [74,75]. Hypernatremia associated with frequent vomiting decreases the biological efficacy of basal as well as stimulated secretion of AVP [77]. (v) Migraine may regress or worsen at the menopause [91]. Restoration of the post-menopausal lost inhibitory opioid tonus with estrogen [91,92] may reduce AVP secretion [49]. (vi) Migraine preventive action of propranolol is neither dose-related nor predictable [2,46,47]; some patients respond to small doses (10-20 mg twice daily) while others require a full β-blocking regimen [93]. Few migraine patients maintain long-term effective remissions with propranolol therapy – a common clinical experience. Paradoxically, propranolol blocks basal and stimulated relase of AVP [94]. *The migraine-preventive effect of propranolol is neither dose-dependent nor evident in all migraineurs, the basis for which remains inexplicable. Suppression of AVP bioavailablity by propranolol might limit its utility in preventing migraine attacks.*

Apomorphine, a powerful and rapid pharmacologic *emetogenic* agent, reduces the frequency and severity of migraine attacks when infused continuously for three weeks, reflecting its prophylactic anti-migraine influence [95] (table 1). Besides, interictal apomorphine blocked the photoparoxysmal EEG response in a patient of migraine with typical aura [96]. Further, in a study of apomorphine inbetween migraine attacks, a striking clinical *dissociation* between headache and nausea and/or vomiting of migraine has been noted; headache was not observed at either the lower or the higher dose (2-10 micrograms/kg, subcutaneously) [97]. Finally, apomorphine-induced nausea/vomiting leads to a striking release of AVP (from 0.9 +/- 0.2 pmol/l to 249 +/- 104 pmol/l at 15 min after the onset of symptoms) in man; on the occasions nausea was not precipitated, apomorphine did not stimulate AVP release [48,50,98,99]. Such AVP release appears to be mediated by dopaminergic stimulation; in seven symptomatic human subjects, the dopamine antagonist haloperidol completely blocked apomorphine-induced AVP release [48]. Remarkably, vomiting (spontaneous) as well as the chemical emetogenic influence of apomorphine can attenuate / abort or prevent migraine headache; AVP appears to play the central role in both clinical situations. In striking contrast to apomorphine (non-selective dopamine *agonist*), metoclopramide (dopamine *antagonist)* is finding use in the management of acute migraine attacks [97,98]. Metoclopramide, like apomorphine, induces a striking release of AVP [100,101]. Muscarinic cholinergic stimulation appears to be the final common pathway for pharmacologically stimulated release of AVP [102,103]. Dopamine receptor hypersensitivity seems to prevail in migraine patients, as manifested by the frequency of occurrence of nausea and/or vomiting, hypotension and yawning, either spontaneously or induced by dopamine agonists at doses that do not affect non-migraine patients [104]; the biological nature of this brain neuronal hypersensitivity is likely to be adaptive rather than pathogenetic (discussed further).

Severe nausea and/or vomiting is often accompanied with altered ANS activity such as hypersalivation, defaecation, skin pallor, increased perspiration, anorexia, and occasionally hypotension and bradycardia (vasovagal syndrome). Stimulation of the vagus nerve in certain species produces a reduction in intraocular pressure (IOP) attributable to concomitant fall in systemic blood pressure [105]. Moreover, in contrast to intracerebroventricular injection, intravenous administration of AVP (but not desmopressin) lowers the IOP [106]. Contrary to the general impression, of the three divisions of the trigeminal nerve, the ophthalmic division (V 1) is the most likely component involved in migraine [19]. A subtle link prevails between migraine, systemic blood pressure, and IOP [19,107], as discussed further in this article. *The development of relatively early nausea and/or vomiting during migraine attacks may be teleologically designed to lower the IOP and increase AVP bioavailability*. The overall biologic importance of this facet of migraine pathophysiology cannot be overemphasized as vomiting is *not* a feature of other primary headaches -- in particular the very severe pain of cluster headache -- as well as of hypertensive headaches (discussed further).

Table 1. AVP and clinical modulators of migraine [37]

Migraine aborting/remitting factors/agents -- ↑ AVP release/bioavailability

Nausea / vomiting
Sleep
Amitriptyline and other tricyclic antidepressants
Smoking / nicotine
Physical exercise
Pregnancy – II and III trimesters
Advancing age
Fluid overload / relative hyponatremia
Apomorphine (dopamine *agonist*)
Metoclopramide (dopamine *antagonist*)
Brain neuronal muscarinic / dopaminergic activation / hypersensitivity
Estrogen

Migraine precipitating factors / agents -- ↓ AVP release / bioavailability

Fear / anxiety-related stress
Alcohol
Reserpine
Vasopressinase (placental)
Hypernatremia – vomiting of pregnancy
Menopause – estrogen replacement -- restoration of lost opioid tonus
Propranolol (patients with failure of prophylaxis)

Key: AVP – arginine vasopressin; ↓-- decrease ; ↑ -- increase.

Vomiting is under control of two functionally distinct medullary centres: the vomiting centre and the chemoreceptor trigger zone of the area postrema. How are the medullary vomiting centres stimulated during migraine attacks? Vomiting (and other 'vegetative' symptoms) of migraine are believed to be stimulated by 5-HT (or other neurally active agents) penetrating the central nervous system (CNS) through specialized brain regions without a blood-brain barrier (BBB), such as the area postrema [38]. However, clinical states of peripheral/systemic or brain neuronal 5-HT excess like carcinoid tumors/syndrome [108] or serotonin syndrome [109], respectively, have not been associated with nausea and/or vomiting. Relief of migraine attacks following vomiting [44-46,51,52] indicates a biological dissociation between migrainous headache and nausea/vomiting, as discussed earlier in this chapter. *Very likely, a physiological mechanism distinct from the origin of the migrainous aura or the headache operates for the genesis of nausea and/or vomiting.* There is also a pathophysiological overlap between migraine, vertigo, and motion sickness [110-112], three illnesses that are characterized by nausea and/or vomiting as a prominent manifestation. Headache, however, is not a major accompaniment of either vertigo or motion sickness. In one study, pathological nystagmus has been seen in over two-third of patients with acute migrainous vertigo [112]. Predominance of the role of visual stimuli and nystagmus (induced by either optokinetic or vestibular stimulation or both) in the pathogenesis of motion sickness has been recently underscored [113]. Repetitive contractions of the extraocular muscles during nystagmus can suddenly generate proprioceptive as well as potentially algogenic afferent orthodromic neural traffic in the ophthalmic division of the trigeminal nerve (V1) in some migraine patients [113]. Rapidly augmented afferent neural traffic to the brain stem might be directed along the nucleus of spinal tract of the trigeminal nerve with 'spillover' to the proximate medullary vomiting centres in those migraine patients who commonly experience nausea and/or vomiting during attacks, and, in most patients with vertigo or motion sickness. Recurrent vomiting with frequent migraine attacks or with the CVS may create a facilitated functional neural pathway at the level of the brain stem through neuronal memory to rapidly effect such 'spillover'. The fact that vomiting usually ameliorates migraine headache indicates that such neural traffic 'spillover' in the brain stem has an adaptive function.

Besides the migraine-stress connection, anticipatory vomiting is a well-known adaptive response to stress [114]. The major subset of migraine-associated CVS [41] possibly represents another form of anticipatory vomiting; stress-induced CVS, with or without headache, may constitute part of the adaptive-avoidance response in some patients [52]. Absence of headache as a prominent feature in CVS again indicates a striking pathogenetic *dissociation* between the two phenomena. Remarkably, plasma AVP elevation is also seen in cluster headache; AVP elevation precedes the onset of the attack and peaks during the attack [115]. Characteristically, vomiting is not a feature of cluster headache [116] although the syndrome is one of the worst painful human experiences that can cause extreme restlessness and drive patients to practice several forms of self-trauma including insertion of sharp or blunt objects between upper teeth or into the nose, compression of the affected eye with a finger, thumb or fist, or rarely suicidal ideation or even suicide [117,118]. Pre-headache rise of AVP in cluster headache also suggests an anticipatory 'learned' adaptive role for AVP release unrelated to the occurrence of nausea and/or vomiting. Although pre-headache levels of AVP have not yet been measured in migraine, given the extended prodrome (also discussed in chapter 5) that might last for several hours or days

[13,36,46,119], the timing of such measurements is practically difficult. Nevertheless, in patients with frequent migraine attacks it is logical to expect activation of secondary adaptive physiological mechanisms that help patients to cope somehow with the morbidity associated with recurrent painful attacks. An anticipatory adaptive role for AVP in migraine is also supported by the report of the attack-preventive effect of AVP; in an open clinical study, 41% of migraine patients reported reduced frequency and intensity of headache attacks during a parenteral prophylactic course of AVP [120]. Further, the anti-migraine potential of metoclopramide probably also involves release of AVP [102,103,121]. Moreover, increased platelet AVP receptors in the attack-free period in the face of normal plasma AVP levels with greater sensitivity in female migraine patients [122,123] also indicates the adaptive nature of the alteration [37]. On the other hand, in a study of chocolate-induced migraine, significant alterations of plasma AVP levels were not detected; Peatfield, Hampton and Grant concluded that AVP does not have an etiological role in migraine [124]. While chocolate has been subsequently disproved as a method for inducing migraine (see chapter 5), the validity of the secondary-reactive or adaptive role of AVP release as well as of platelet aggregability in migraine pathophysiology (further discussed in chapter 9) is not affected by this single, open, study of six patients. Intriguingly, intravenous injection of AVP results in vomiting and retching in humans [125] and in dogs [126]; the emetogenic effect of low doses of exogenous (peripheral) AVP probably involves central effects [127]. *A direct role for centrally-released AVP in precipitating nausea and/or vomiting in migraine patients cannot be excluded.*

In summary, nausea and/or vomiting appears to subserve an important biologically adaptive function in migraine. Early nausea and/or vomiting in migraine might be telelogically designed to release AVP and to lower IOP. Central mechanisms [anticipatory, pre-migraine headache neuroendocrine (AVP) and / or V 1 orthodromic neural 'spillover' in the brain stem] might be involved in the triggering of the nausea and/or vomiting reflex during migraine attacks. There appears to be sufficient theoretical background to begin to conceive of a fundamental pathophysiological dissociation between the mechanistic origins of the aura or headache (or both) and that of the nausea and/or vomiting of migraine attacks [128].

Teleology is the unfashionable lady without whom no biologist can live, yet he is ashamed to show himself with her in public – Ernst Wilhelm von Brücke(1819-1892).

Chapter 4

MAGNESIUM DEPLETION, MIGRAINE, AND CELLULAR ADAPTATION

Science is not a particular set of techniques; it is, rather, a state of mind, or attitude, and the organizational conditions which allow that attitude to be expressed. – N. Mays, C. Pope [Br Med J. 1995;311:109-112]

Migraine might be regarded as the prototypic magnesium depletion-related photosensitive headache [129]. A systemic and brain magnesium deficit prevails in migraine patients between attacks (headache-free periods). As reviewed [129], heterogenous and inconsistent decreases in intra- or extra-cellular total or ionized magnesium concentrations in serum, saliva, erythrocytes, mononuclear cells, thrombocyte [130-134] and brain [135-137] have been seen in migraine patients. Oral or intravenous therapeutic supplementation of magnesium under controlled conditions, however, results in unpredictable or unexpectedly negative responses [134-142].

The basis for clinical efforts directed at experimental magnesium supplementation for treatment (both preventive and abortive) of migraine stems from the belief that low levels of magnesium in the brain of migraine patients represent a *pathogenetic* deficiency. The state of brain magnesium ionic (Mg^{2+}) homeostasis is believed to be a key feature in the putative migraine pathogenetic cascade related to central or brain neuronal hyperexcitability [9,12,17,18]. Critical limitations to a pathogenetic role for magnesium deficiency/depletion in migraine, however, include: (i) Mg^{2+} depletion or deficiency is not specific to migraine; (ii) it is unknown why migraine patients should spontaneously become Mg^{2+} depleted (during exacerbations) or repleted (during remissions); and (iii) no systemic influence can explain either lateralizing (unilateral, bilateral, or side-shifting) migraine headache or post-stress headache [36,144,145]. A greater degree of

Mg^{2+} deficiency has been seen in patients with tension-type headache and cluster headache [142,145]; a primary pathogenetic role for Mg^{2+} depletion/deficiency has not been conceived for these primary headache variants. Also, the inconsistent migraine attack-aborting action of magnesium supplementation is not specific to migraine; in a case-control study, intravenous magnesium supplementation appears to offer rapid relief in cluster headache [142].

The range of pathologies associated with Mg deficiency / depletion is staggering [146]. Widely diverse clinical conditions and circumstances linked only by the common thread of stress, acute or chronic, manifest magnesium deficiency [143,146,147]. *A redistribution of magnesium from plasma into soft tissues or bones can occur acutely in such situations*. Hypomagnesemia is often found in hospitalized inpatients (65% of those in intensive care and up to 12% of those on general wards); diabetes mellitus is the most common cause of hypomagnesemia probably secondary to osmotic diuresis [146,147]. Remarkably, hypoglycemia -- but not hyperglycemia -- has been associated with migraine [13,46,82]. Magnesium deficiency is found in patients with non-migrainous headaches, 30% of patients with alcoholism admitted to hospitals, hypertension, pancreatitis, extensive burns, profuse sweating, chronic diuresis, acute myocardial infarction, premenstrual syndrome, and many other varied conditions. In all clinical states with magnesium depletion or hypomagnesemia, brain Mg^{+2} will also be lowered. *No study has compared the levels of brain Mg^{2+} of patients with migraine against those in significantly stressful clinical situations but without migrainous headache* [143]. Also, except for premenstrual syndrome, migraine has not been particularly linked to any of the several known causes of magnesium deficiency [143]. Further, alcohol ingestion, not hospitalization of patients with alcoholism or abstinence, is associated with migraine [143]. Finally, magnesium is a *vasodilator* and a competitive calcium-antagonist [139,141]. Nitroglycerin, a powerful vasodilator and experimental model for migraine, commonly precipitates typical headache attacks – but not aura -- in migraine patients [148]. Administration of a vasodilating agent like magnesium during migraine attacks is a counterintuitive therapeutic strategy that challenges logical thinking. As a self-limited disorder, nevertheless, spontaneous resolution of migraine attacks can never be excluded in clinical trials; interpretation of results of migraine-abortive therapies – in particular, vasodilators -- must, therefore, always be guarded.

A cellular-level adaptive function for the cardiac myocyte has been advanced for *hypomagnesemia* in the rapidly-changing frequently fatal milieu of pump failure in acute myocardial infarction [149]. For several decades, the scientific rationale for magnesium supplementation in patients with acute myocardial infarction appeared logical and secure [150]. This belief arose from experimental models as well as clinical experience; attenuation of reperfusion injury and free radical damage, and, improved myocardial energy status were some of the perceived benefits. Despite a seemingly defensible theoretical background including favorable meta-analysis for use of an inexpensive agent like magnesium for myocardial salvage, controlled clinical trials did not support such a therapeutic strategy [151,152]. In a rare reversal of theoretical principles, the clinical futility of routine magnesium supplementation in acute myocardial infarction was finally disproved in a RCT [153,154]. Magnesium supplementation in acute myocardial infarction effects a triple-inotropic myocardial jeopardy and worsens pump function, the most critical determinant of survival in this clinical situation [149]. Such reversal of an apparently defensible theoretical foundation as well as clinically secure body of evidence was possible only because the end point (mortality) was very sharply defined [26].

The theoretical basis for prophylactic or abortive magnesium supplementation in primary headaches including migraine is much more ambiguous; also, small effects of treatment and use of soft end-points in pain research (such as frequency or intensity of migraine headaches) invalidate the results of most RCTs [26]. More importantly, transport of magnesium from blood to cerebrospinal fluid (CSF) across the intact BBB is limited in normal humans; even intravenous administration of magnesium sulphate does not increase CSF magnesium concentration [155]. In the absence of significant disruption of the BBB, therefore, orally or intravenously administered Mg cannot critically affect brain neuronal function (or CSD) [156].

Hypomagnesemia – whether part of deficiency or depletion-related dysregulation of the magnesium status – appears to be an important physiologically-adaptive mechanism that enables optimal operation of a host of calcium-dependent cellular level functions during acute or chronic stress or life-threatening conditions. Clinically, the most dramatic negative effect of magnesium supplementation in human beings has been seen with decreased survival in acute myocardial infarction. Remarkably, although magnesium sulphate is now the drug of choice for both the prevention and the treatment of eclampsia, the mode of its rather unpredictable anti-convulsant action is still unclear [157,158]. Blockade of brain N-methyl-D-aspartate receptors by exogenously administered magnesium [18,159] is an attractive concept for which there is but little evidence in humans. Intriguingly, exogenous magnesium itself attenuates enhanced BBB permeability in different experimental models [160-163], rendering quite unlikely the possibility of any direct protective action (of administered magnesium) on brain neuronal hyper-activity during migraine attacks or inbetween attacks. Finally, basal levels of free Mg^{2+} in the CSF are threefold that in plasma while the walls of the cerebral arteries have almost double the content of Mg seen in systemic arteries [164]. These peculiarities of brain magnesium metabolism help to understand why access of exogenous magnesium into the CSF-CNS is so tightly regulated. In effect, higher intrinsic or basal CSF as well as mural cerebral arterial magnesium levels appear to offer a degree of natural or spontaneous brain neuronal protection from 'hyper-activation' (a form of neuronal dampening) in disease as well as in health.

In summary, therapeutically administered exogenous magnesium – oral or intravenous -- probably does not significantly or critically influence brain neuronal function. As magnesium is a competitive calcium-antagonist at the cellular level, hypomagnesemia would optimize calcium-dependent cranial vasoconstriction – intracranial or extracranial or both -- in migraine patients during attacks. Magnesium, in general, also opposes release of catecholamines from the adrenal gland [165], another facet of the finely balanced homeostatic system governing vascular integrity and antinociception in the face of cranial vasodilatory antidromic V1 activation (discussed further in Chapter 5). Hypomagnesemia or magnesium depletion in migraine patients very likely represents an important adaptive feature (table 3). Magnesium supplementation appears to have no scientifically-supported role in management of migraine.

Our organs always improvise means of meeting every new situation...The body perceives the remote as well as the near, the future as well as the present.
– Alexis Carrel (1873-1944).

Chapter 5

STRESS AND MIGRAINE: BRAIN AUTONOMIC FUNCTION, BP, IOP, AND BBB

The mind clearly plays a part in the pathogenesis of migraine.[1] Equally clearly, we do not know how the mind brings about the migraine attack.

One of the few clinical absolutes that can offer definitive insight into migraine mechanisms is the temporal relation of stress to occurrence of migraine attacks. As mentioned previously, the term 'stress' itself has little meaning in terms of understanding any illness, including migraine [32,33]. 'Post-stress' headache, 'weekend migraine' or 'let-up phenomenon' or 'shopping headache' are descriptive catch phrases that serve more to cloak our ignorances rather than to shed light on causal mechanisms [166]. What these terms do indicate is that migraine commonly develops well after maximal impact of the attack precipitant. Additionally, the emphasis on studying the clinical phenomenology of migraine prodrome or postdrome for clues to its pathogenesis [166,167] has hitherto yielded little further clarification. Coining of new words rarely adds to pathophysiological insight. While it may no longer be fashionable in migraine research lexicon to use the term 'prophylaxis', the substitutive in-vogue term 'prevention' has added but little to overall comprehension of the entity. Turning to refinements of language is an intrinsic human tendency in science as well as in politics; in both fields, such 'advances' do not herald any incremental insight. *Protagonists of CSD have neither attempted to link post-stress migraine attacks to CSD nor ever acknowledged their failure to do so.*

Stress is the commonest known precipitant of migraine attacks [13, 17, 31, 82]. Not only is the causal link or mechanistic relation between migraine and stress unknown, common occurrence of 'post-stress headache' suggests that stress

---

[1] J.N. Blau. Lancet 1994;344:1623-1624.

has a limited protective effect in most migraine patients.[33,36,37] Excitement with a step-up in intrinsic brain noradrenergic (and very likely serotonergic and cholinergic) activity (also see Chapters 8, 9) can swiftly end or abort an ongoing migraine attack. In a well-documented case, General Ulysses Grant's migraine headache following a mostly sleepless night dramatically resolved when he received the surrender note from the messenger of the Confederate General Robert E. Lee in the American Civil War.[168,169] In his memoirs, Grant recalled that he felt no exultation on Lee's surrender. He felt "sad and depressed" and "like anything rather than rejoicing at the downfall of a foe who had fought so long and valiantly, and had suffered so much for a cause".[169] Surge or step-up in brain noradrenergic activity (overt or subconscious / subliminal) is a common accompaniment of stress-related arousal regardless of complexity of feelings or perceptions (whether immediate or a delayed after-reflection). Both 'post-stress headache' and amelioration or relief of ongoing migraine headache with augmentation of stress underscore the *protective* nature of intrinsic brain noradrenergic activation.

Neither the headache nor the visual or sensory aura preceding it marks the true beginning of a migraine attack; these symptoms are only part of an evolving process and represent the end-points of a series of physiologic changes.[170] Till very recently, it has not been possible to translate this rationalizing observation into neurophysiologic and neuroendocrine templates. The interval between exposure to the headache-provoking stimulus or clinical circumstance and the onset of prodromal symtoms might be termed as the 'pre-prodromal' phase of migraine.[171] Although the onset of migraine, strictly (and appropriately) is with the 'pre-prodromal phase' [22], current pathogenetic theories do not reflect this fundamental aspect. The prodromal phase (premonitory symptoms) of migraine itself is variable and can extend from several hours to several days. [13,46,47,119,170] The primary pathogenetic aberration that underlies migraine actually begins with the 'pre-prodromal' phase.[22,171]

Significance of the 'pre-prodromal' phase of migraine can be analysed by the substantial delay in onset of migraine attacks in the following clinical circumstances: (i) stress; (ii) exercise; (iii) ingestion of alcohol, with the patient waking up with a 'hangover' or migraine headache next morning [13]; (ii) ingestion of tyramine containing foods, involving a delay upto 22 hours [172]; cocaine abuse or abstinence [173,174]; caffeine withdrawal over the weekend [175]; exposure to m-chlorophenylpiperazine (m-CPP) [176]; and nitroglycerin ingestion or infusion [148]. Primary headache associated with catastrophic psychological (non-physical) trauma [177] or physical trauma [178] is similarly associated with a significant delay in onset. Delay in onset of attacks of MA+ or

MA- encompasses the 'pre-prodromal' and prodromal phases of migraine and is completely analogous to the period after an 'acute injury'[34] during which the migraine subject remains largely unaware of the threat of impending painful cephalic disturbance and continues to function appropriately.[36] In other words, the variable period between acute physical injury to any part of the body (cuts, fractures, or amputations) and onset of pain in up to 37% of patients who were neither distracted nor in shock [34] parallels the significant time interval between exposure to the headache-provoking stimulus and onset of migraine attack, during which period a host of adaptive physiological processes are activated and operate efficiently to keep the attack (aura or headache or both) at bay. The physiological system(s) primarily affected in migraine and post-traumatic headache, therefore, must necessarily be afforded a considerable (but limited and exhaustible) degree of protection by homeostatic defense mechanisms, thereby allowing the subject to continue to function normally for some time despite the stressful stimulus or situation; this protection is obviously unlimited or inexhaustible in the majority of the general population who are *not* susceptible to headaches. Such adaptive reaction is liable to fatigue variably in different migraine patients as well as in the same migraine patient on different occasions; onset of migraine (acute attack or chronic daily headache) possibly represents overwhelming or fatigue of this adaptive 'system'.[33,36,37] Also, most migraine patients continue to function during the attack (after onset of aura or pain or both), again extending the analogy with acute injury in animals and man. 37%-70% of wounded subjects continue to function in the period after acute injury; such adaptation is the outcome of a meticulously-orchestrated parallel activation of multiple physiological (secondary stress or reactive/adaptive) processes.[34]

Historically, migraine research has been characterized by a series of serendipitous therapeutic events that have channeled thinking of researchers and coloured perception of primary headache therapists over the last several decades. Advent of β-blockers [179], scalp injection of botulinum toxin [180], and closure of patent foramen ovale (PFO) / atrial septal defect (ASD) [181], are major chance events influencing current migraine theory and therapy. Serendipity in medical therapeutics (cart-before-the-horse) can be a double-edged sword that extracts hidden but heavy costs in terms of delayed comprehension of disease mechanisms, perpetuation of medical myths or therapeutic empiricism, and justification for interventional misadventures. Approximately forty years ago, the chance discovery of the migraine preventive effect of β-blockers ostensibly marks a research milestone. While empiric use of propranolol has become established as a 'gold standard' in preventive migraine therapeutics and has provided much needed but unpredictable, partial and dose-unrelated symptomatic relief to many patients, it also generated the corollary that intrinsic or brain sympathetic nervous system (SNS) hyperfunction must exert a deleterious and pathogenetic influence. Despite the generally accepted adaptive / protective role ('alarm' or 'stress' response) of the SNS during 'fright', 'flight', or 'fight' [182], this corollary finally crystallized the common perception of neuroscientists in the later half of the twentieth century as the biobehavioral model of migraine [17] -- a frequently cited article underlying much research efforts over the last two decades. Although Welch candidly acknowledged that the postulated pathogenetic role for intrinsic brain nodrenergic activation was speculative [17], the biobehavioral model of migraine struck a chord of consensus among neurologists devoted to migraine research and forms the conceptual bedrock of much of the current evidence as well as of the extrapolation regarding brain neuronal hyperfunction as the central or key event in genesis of migraine attacks. *Desperate for a respectable brain-theory that would substantiate the long-held concept that migraine was a brain neuronal disorder, otherwise overly-critical neurologists refused both to see or recognize the yawning gaps in the biobehavioral model as well as to put the theory to the searing test of logic – a classic example of herd mentality among scientists. In this unwieldy process, the adaptive role of the ANS / SNS mutated into a pathogenetic process, eventually gaining the virtually immutable status of dogma etched in stone .*

Sympathetic dysfunction in migraine patients has been noted in a variety of diagnostic tests and through clinical signs by many investigators for over 150 years [31] and has been confirmed in a recent population-based study [183]. During headache-free periods, migraine patients have a reduction in sympathetic function compared to no-migraine patients as seen in functional tests of the SNS and clinical data; as a chronic disorder of SNS but with an anatomically intact SNS, a parallel might be seen between migraine on the one hand and pure autonomic failure and multiple system atrophy on the other.[31] NE-related functions, a direct 'online' measure of SNS activity [184], appear particularly affected in migraine.[31] A review of five published reports of supine plasma NE levels in migraine patients during headache-free periods showed lower NE levels than in controls, ranging from 41% - 91% (average 61%) of matched control values.[31] Following an orthostatic change in headache-free migraine patients, rise of plasma NE was 46-74% (average 59%) lower than in matched controls. [31] The important unresolved issue is whether or not such SNS dysfunction is pathogenetic [31] or otherwise. Nevertheless, it has been suggested that migraine attacks occur due to reciprocal alterations in NE (decreased release following exhaustion / depletion of neural stores) and dopamine, adenosine and prostaglandin (increased release) after prolonged or excessive SNS stimulation.

[31] A balanced overview of available evidences, however, does not support a pathogenetic role for dopamine in migraine.[185] *With both dopamine agonists (apomorphine) and antagonists (metoclopramide) being able to abort / attenuate migraine attacks (Table 1), dopamine and dopaminergic phenomena in migraine are highly unlikely to have significant pathogenetic influence. In migraine research, unfortunately, from time to time, a key pathogenetic influence has been attributed to several different individual neuro-peptides.* ***In-vivo, neuro-peptides do not work in splendid isolation but in an extremely well-organized counter-balancing fashion. Laboratory medicine is intrinsically reductionist.*[13]** ***The exclusive focus on one or two factors creates an artificial individuality, dividing the whole into parts that seem to have a life of their own and are more often than not irreconcilable.*[2,3]**

While SNS hypofunction in the laboratory is not as consistent or pervasive as one might hope or expect, given the unambiguous adaptive role of the SNS, theories that directly implicate the ANS in pathogenesis of migraine are counterintuitive and work against teleologic fundamentals.[33,36] Remarkably, in the only pre-headache (prodromal or, more accurately, 'pre-prodromal') study of catecholamines in migraine patients, plasma total catecholamines and specifically plasma NE were significantly higher in the 3 hours before the subjects awoke with migraine.[186] The immediate pre-headache phase of migraine is, therefore, clearly associated with catecholamine excess and peripheral sympathoadrenal activation.[33] Also, it is conceptually confusing to extrapolate low catecholamine values seen during headache-free intervals to pathogenesis of migraine attacks. [33] More importantly, β-blockers do not generally restore or elevate plasma NE levels but characteristically augment peripheral adrenergic hypersensitivity (Raynaud's phenomenon). β-blockers, thus, pharmacologically replicate precisely the same changes as have been noted in the peripheral SNS in headache-free migraine patients.[33] Additionally, propranolol and other β-blockers useful in migraine prevention do not reverse or correct the putative SNS disturbance (hypofunction) regarded by many investigators as a primary and pathogenetic feature of migraine; conversely, ß-blockers induce or worsen SNS hypofunction. [33] Next, despite their hypotensive effect, β-blockers or calcium antagonists generally do not replicate or aggravate orthostatic / relative hypotension-related symptoms commonly seen by several investigators in untreated migraine patients in a variety of situations such as after standing, after tilting, after Valsalva

---

[2] V.K. Gupta. Cephalalgia 1994;14:411-412.

[3] "In fact, we divide a whole into parts. And we are astonished that the parts, thus separated, exactly fit each other when they are put together again by our mind" – A. Carrel. Man, The Unknown. Hamish Hamilton Ltd., London, 1959.

maneuver or during the hand-grip test.[33] Moreover, dopamine receptor hypersensitivity prevails in migraine patients, as demonstrated by induction of yawning, nausea, vomiting, hypotension, and other symptoms of a migraine attack by dopaminergic agonists (such as bromocriptine) at doses that do not affect non-migraine patients.[104] *Central dopamine hypersensitivity in migraine patients might indicate an adaptive readiness of the vasopressinergic system (discussed previously) rather than a pathogenetic aberration.*

There appears to be a strong link between migraine prevention, low systemic blood pressure, and low IOP [19]: (i) Amitriptyline – an established migraine preventive drug [2] that induces central noradrenergic, serotonergic, and vasopressinergic activation (see Chapter 9) -- produces postural hypotension to a statistically significant degree.[187] Although glaucoma is a contraindication for therapy with amitriptyline, only one case of acute congestive gluacoma has been reported following amitriptyline overdose.[188] Despite common use of amitriptyline for migraine prevention over several decades, acute congestive glaucoma has not been reported in a single migraine patient; the relatively low-doses that are used for migraine prevention probably do not allow development of this complication. Protriptyline, a member of the tricyclic family, potentiates adrenergic activity and actually lowers IOP when administered topically.[189] (ii) Serotonergic antagonists – methysergide and cypropheptadine, other known migraine preventive agents [2] (see Chapter 9 for further references) – lower central serotonergic or peripheral renal sympathetic nervous discharge, respectively, and tend to lower the blood pressure experimentally.[190,191] Also, despite the possibility of precipitating acute congestive glaucoma due to mydriasis (class effect for anti-histamines), common use of cyproheptadine for childhood migraine prevention [2] (also see Chapter 9) indicates that, at least in migraine patients, the potential glaucomatous or ocular hypertensive effect of cyprophetadine is a largely theoretical issue. (iii) Methysergide inhibits calcitonin-gene related peptide (CGRP)-induced vasodilatation, increase in IOP, and breakdown of blood-aqueous barrier in the rabbit.[192] Although the species difference must be underscored, methysergide and cyproheptadine both tend to lower systemic blood pressure and IOP. (iv) Topical verapamil induces sustained reduction of IOP in ocular hypertension without systemic cardiovascular changes. [193] In contrast to the clinical utility of verapamil [194-196], nifedipine has not been found useful for migraine prevention.[197] Despite a prominent systemic hypotensive action, nifedipine has no effect on IOP in humans.[198] (v) Bromocriptine lowers IOP in normal volunteers even without changing the blood pressure.[199] (vi) Several other migraine preventive drugs – with established or limited evidence for prophylactic value -- reduce blood pressure as well as IOP

[19,105] (Table 2). *Given the link between systemic blood pressure, headache, and IOP [200] as well as the possible etiologic link between ocular choroidal blood flow-IOP and migraine [19], the tendency to maintain low blood pressure between migraine attacks likely constitutes an important peripheral adaptive mechanism designed to maintain a low basal ocular chroidal blood flow and IOP.* In general, pharmacological agents and clinical states associated with a relatively low blood pressure are accompanied by lower IOP.

Although the exact pathophysiological role of relative hypotension in migraine patients during headache-free periods is presently unknown, closure of ASD can dramatically and immediately precipitate or aggravate attacks of MA+ or MA- without any alteration of brain noradrenergic function or possible link to CSD; such aggravation of migraine sometimes manifests a prominent circadian pattern.[201-203] Several important gaps remain in the postulated etiologic link between PFO/ASD and migraine [181,204-208] (see Chapter 11). Closure of uncomplicated atrial septal defects, nevertheless, increases left ventricular stroke volume; this cardiovascular effect of ASD-closure or its effect on circadian variation of the stroke volume, pulsatile ocular choroidal blood flow, and IOP might be one variable underlying sudden post-procedure worsening of the migrainous diathesis.[181,204-208] Aggravation of migraine attacks after ASD-closure generally subsides after a few months; cardiovascular *acclimatization* and ocular *tissue creep* are possibly involved.[204,207]

The failure of β-blockers with intrinsic sympathomimetic activity such as pindolol, oxprenolol, alprenolol, and acebutolol to offer significant migraine prophylaxis has not been rationalized [209-212] and remains a vexing enigma. As partial sympathomimetic agents / agonists, such β-blockers must affect some basic cardio- and cranio-vascular function that aggravates the tendency to develop migraine. Remarkably, in striking contrast to propranolol, pindolol *increases* heart rate and cardiac output.[213] In such clinical states – similar to post-ASD closure – cardiac stroke volume and pulsatile choroidal blood flow / IOP both are likely to increase. Additionally, patients with comorbid migraine and panic disorder have a longer duration of panic disorder, a higher number of attacks and a heavier family loading for panic disorder and headache.[214] The link between anxiety / panic states and migraine [214,215] may be based, besides active suppression of AVP secretion (discussed previously, Chapter 3), on similar underlying cardiovascular pathophysiology. Anxiety states are associated with the following cardiac variables: enhanced myocardial contractility, less afterload, bigger preload, bigger stroke volume and cardiac output, and higher blood pressure.[216] In addition, clinical states with prolonged autonomic arousal can be associated with largely unpredictable exhaustion of the ANS or the vasopressinergic system or both, that can, in turn, set the stage for occurrence of migraine. SNS hypofunction in migraine patients between attacks likely maintains low cardiac contractility, low left ventricular stroke volume and cardiac output, low blood pressure as well as relatively diminished cranial and ocular choroidal blood flow and IOP; while most migraine preventive pharmacological agents effect such systemic and ocular hemodynamic change, several clinical states associated with migraine periodically and transiently effect the opposite physiological state (Table 2). Documentation of such alterations at the level of the eye is fraught with difficulties. Even with home tonometry, transient elevations of IOP are very difficult to measure.(107) *In the postulated link between migraine and the eye, it is the choroidal blood flow and the corneo-scleral stretch / elasticity / rigidity that are primarily involved. In this context, IOP becomes a surrogate (but rather unrepresentative) marker of the slow-order fluctuations of ocular hemodynamics.* **There is a fundamental difference between glaucoma (including primary open angle glaucoma) and the ocular hemodynamic aberration proposed for migraine. Furthermore, the postulated ocular hemodynamic disturbance develops in the 'pre-prodromal' phase, at a time when the migraine patient is asymptomatic.**

The second key theoretical misdirection that followed the serendipitous discovery of migraine preventive effect of propranolol involves confusion about role of the parasympathetic nervous system (PNS). Changes in ANS functions recorded during migraine attacks have been uncertainly attributed to autonomic dysregulation or imbalance between SNS and PNS.[223] Presently, it is uncertain whether PNS *hypofunction* or *hyperfunction* prevails during migraine attacks; also the role of the PNS between migraine attacks as well as in the pre-attack phase is vague.[224,225]

Prolongation of cardiac PR-(atrio-ventricular conduction) interval,[223] delayed gastric emptying / gastric stasis ('pylorospasm'), and pupillary miosis dissociated from ptosis but persisting between migraine attacks (see Chapter 6) indicate prevalence of generalized parasympathetic overactivity in concert with SNS stimulation.[224,225] A linked conceptually challenging issue is the suggested role of PNS in occurrence of cutaneous allodynia in some migraine patients, and, its presumed link with pathogenetic central and peripheral neuronal sensitization.[226,227,228] One, cutaneous allodynia is not specific to migraine pathophysiology but is, in general, a common non-specific feature of pain neurophysiology in health as well as in disease.[229-233] Two, pain levels are not significantly different between migraine attacks with allodynia or without allodynia,[234] and, on different occasions, the same patient might manifest allodynic or non-allodynic attacks [235]. Three, the parasympathetic neurotransmitter, acetylcholine stimulates AVP release (discussed previously,

Chapter 3) and the antinociceptive action of nicotine and nicotine agonists is rapidly evolving.[236,237] Four, donepezil – a second generation parasympathomimetic central and peripheral antinociceptive cholinesterase inhibitor – readily crosses the BBB, induces dose-dependent antinociception in mice, and offers prophylaxis for MA+ or MA- comparable to propranolol (40 mg b.i.d.).[238] Finally, development of allodynia has been suggested to imply a defect in antinociception in migraine patients.[239] Antinociception, however, is reportedly enhanced during migraine attacks.[128] Fundamentally, the ANS and its two limbs are biologically adaptive; it is illogical to conceive of pathogenetic pathways that directly involve the SNS or the PNS, either singly or jointly. In migraine patients, it is very likely that a secondary reactive / adaptive, parallel, peripheral and central activation of both SNS and PNS develops early in the attacks.

Table 2. Migraine-preventive drugs, blood pressure, and intraocular pressure

Pharmacological agent	Blood pressure	Intra-ocular pressure
Propranolol	↓	↓ (O, T, I)
Atenolol	↓	↓ (O)
Nadolol	↓	↓ (O)
Timolol	↓	↓ (O,T)
Metoprolol	↓	↓ (O,T) [217,218]
Pindolol	↓	↓ (T) [219,220]
Oxprenolol	↓	↓ (T) [220]
Verapamil	↓	↓ (T)
Nifedipine	↓	No effect (O,I) [198]; ↓ (T) [221]
Flunarizine	↓	↓ [221]
Cyproheptadine	↓	↓ (experimental evidence); CI – angle closure glaucoma (mydriatic class effect for anti-histamines)
Methysergide	↓	↓ (experimental evidence)
Amitriptyline	↓	? / ↓ (Class effect) [189]
Mianserin [304]	? ↓ [308]	?
Bromocriptine	↓	↓
Donepezil	? / ↓ (overdose)	↓ (O,T) [222]
Melatonin [340]	?	↓ [338]

Key: ↓ -- decrease; ↑ -- increase; CI – contraindicated; ? – unknown/uncertain; O – oral administration; T – topical administration; I – intravenous administration.

The third key conceptual diversion that followed the serendipitous discovery of migraine prophylactic role of propranolol involves the BBB. In a striking paradox, the current thrust in migraine therapeutics -- with the industry-sponsored but speculative 'migraine-preventive' role for triptans – almost completely ignores the role of BBB penetrability of anti-migraine agents. In brain-related pharmacokinetics, nevertheless, the ability of potentially beneficial drugs to readily or freely cross the intact BBB is a given basic absolute. Unlike migraine abortive agents, effective migraine prophylactic agents must modulate the 'afferent' limb or early-phase physiological events.[20] *If -- as is generally presumed -- migraine is indeed consequent to neuronal dysfunction at the level of the brain, all migraine preventive agents must freely or readily cross the intact BBB in order to critically influence brain neuronal function inbetween attacks* (see Chapter 4). Certain research events and trends have, unfortunately, encouraged the thinking that the BBB is unimportant in analyses of migraine preventive pharmacotherapy. Absence of any discernible pharmacokinetic pattern in the migraine preventive effect of various β-blockers in relation to the BBB suggested that brain penetrability was of little consequence; oxprenolol and alprenolol both penetrate into the CNS but do not show migraine-preventive activity [209]. Nevertheless, approximately a quarter century ago, the fact that atenolol can prevent both MA+ or MA- attacks as effectively as propranolol was regarded as a curious, rather unsettling, finding as penetration of atenolol into brain tissue is minimal or negligible.[240,241] While the surprise factor has, regrettably, worn off, the consistent efficacy of atenolol in preventing migraine has been re-confirmed in controlled studies and case reports, and, the issue has been critically reviewed.[19-22,242,243,244] Atenolol is currently established as a drug of first choice for migraine prophylaxis [245,246] but does *not* readily cross the BBB or critically alter any brain function possibly related to migraine pathogenesis.[19-22] Nadolol has shown migraine preventive activity comparable to propranolol [246,247,248] but like atenolol, does not freely cross the intact BBB.[209] Verapamil, a widely used prophylactic agent with limited evidence of benefit [2, 194-196] does not cross the BBB.[249] Some therapists prefer to use verapamil prophylactically in patients with migraine aura, with or without headache, particularly when the auras are frequent or associated with hemiparesis [195] although verapamil is not known to affect any brain neuronal function directly. To maintain that migraine is the outcome of a primary aberration of brain neuronal function in the face of confirmed ability of atenolol and nadolol and possibly verapamil to prevent both MA+ and MA- attacks challenges rational thinking.[19-22,144] On the other hand, the recommended use of anti-convulsant drugs for migraine prevention [9,18], although pharmacologically controversial and clinically limited [19-22,250,251], mandates ready penetration of the BBB and access to the CNS of such pharmacological agents in order to critically influence brain neuronal function ('stabilization'). Like atenolol, triptans have only limited brain penetrability and are not known to influence *any* brain neuronal function. The scope of this chapter does not permit a critical discussion of the therapeutic role of anti-epileptics in migraine prevention,[250,251] but in the context of the BBB, these divergent clinico-pharmacological facts cannot be reconciled. Triptans show a non-cranial / non-trigeminal antinociceptive action that is not specific for migraine (see Chapter 2). Again, BBB penetrability is the key factor as this antinociceptive effect is seen only following intra-thecal administration of sumatriptan.[4]

In concert with other clinical and experimental evidences that suggest a peripheral origin, the pharmacological absolute offered by established migraine preventive agents that do not cross the intact BBB questions the long-entrenched belief that migraine originates at the level of the brain or brain stem.[19-22, 25, 144, 156, 250, 251] *While no amount of supportive data ever proves a hypothesis, any hypothesis may be disproved by a single piece of contradictory evidence.*[252] Insofar as the theory of genesis of migraine through central neuronal aberration is concerned, the rarely-discussed but irreconcilable paradox of prophylaxis offered by pharmacological agents that do not cross the intact BBB or critically influence brain neuronal function is indeed such a contradictory evidence. *Currently, few neurologists use atenolol as a first drug or at all for migraine prophylaxis, and, atenolol is also omitted from several authoritative reviews. In direct proportion to its unambiguous, significantly negative impact oncurrent brain-centric theories of migraine pathogenesis, the prophylactic value of atenolol seems almost to be a closely guarded secret. The failure of atenolol to progress from an unexpected 'conceptual inconvenience' to a defining event in evolution of understanding of migraine might be squarely attributed to an overriding but premature philosophic commitment by its researchers.*

The fourth drawback of propranolol-related serendipity in migraine therapeutics relates directly to interpretation of central or brain neuronal (dys)function. The corollary that gained ground implied that stimulated brain / intrinsic central noradrenergic activity plays a central role in the pathogenesis of migraine.[17,18] Although, presently, central / brain sympathetic function is unmeasurable, the key to understanding migraine lies in its indirect and inferential comprehension through relevant clinical and pharmacological features (discussed in part in this section): (i) Caffeine and cocaine *delay* migraine attack onset while

---

[4] T. Nikai, A.I. Basbaum, A.H. Ahn. Pain 2008;139:533-40.

amitriptyline and (dextro)amphetamine offer significant prophylaxis in some migraine (and chronic tension-type headache) patients.[13,31,173-175,253] Caffeine, amitriptyline, and amphetamine unambiguously *stimulate* brain noradrenergic function. Cocaine is a well-established drug of abuse that unarguably and powerfully *stimulates* CNS/brain neuronal function involving alteration and blockade of cellular membrane transport and reuptake inhibition of dopamine, NE, and 5-HT.[254,255] Cocaine enhances intrinsic brain synaptic bioavailability of monoaminines; the adaptive nature of such activation of brain monoaminergic function [254] is highlighted by the fact that headaches following cocaine administration subside immediately with its readministration.[174] Also, unsurprisingly, some patients experiencing chronic headache may begin using cocaine as self-medication for pain.[256] (ii) Amitriptyline has been the drug of choice for chronic pain since 1964 when Lance and Curran showed its efficacy. [257,258] As a group, tricyclic antidepressants show significant analgesic activity while the evidence for selective serotonin reuptake inhibitors is conflicting.[258] Amitriptyline (and other tricyclic antidepressants) -- like cocaine -- inhibits reuptake of both NE as well as 5-HT [258]; increased neuronal availability of NE appears to contribute more prominently towards its analgesic activity. *Although in neuro-psychiatry literature, amitriptyline is clearly acknowledged both as a noradrenergic agonist as well as a serotonergic agonist, in migraine research literature amitrityline was for long erroneously classified as a serotonergic antagonist.* ***Till today, in migraine research, amitriptyline has not been acknowledged as a 5-HT agonist simply because certain known serotonergic antagonists offer some degree of migraine attack prevention. Such juxtaposition of facts would not allow the central / brain serotonin theory of migraine to be maintained.*** (iii) While anticonvulsants appear to have some limited migraine preventive effect [9,17,18,19-22,250,251], both amphetamine and tricyclic antidepressants enhance brain cortical excitability and can induce seizures.[254] ***The fact that both anticonvulsant and pro-convulsant drugs might prevent migraine is, again, logically challenging.*** [19-22,254] (iv) Migraine provoking effect of both tyramine and chocolate has been disproved by nasogastric administration.[259,260] Nevertheless, it is important to underscore that tyramine releases catecholamines (specifically NE) or bradykinin in the tissues [170] while phenylethylamine has been conceptualized as the body's natural amphetamine. [254,261] (v) Lumbar intrathecal administration of NE produces potent analgesia by a profound inhibitory action on spinal nociceptive interneurons while phentolamine when injected similarly with methysergide blocks morphine analgesia, indicating that catecholamines in the CSF naturally promote analgesia.[34] (vi) Delay in onset of migraine attacks in a variety of clinical circumstances, including stress (see above), indicates that, for a variably limited period, subliminal / subconscious brain arousal is protective in nature. *Against this background, it appears quite difficult to maintain a pathogenetic role for brain neuronal dysfunction or for intrinsic CNS norepinephrine aberration in the pathogenesis of migraine.*

In summary, stress-induced SNS and PNS hyperfunction occurs in parallel and is primarily adaptive in nature. Besides migraine attacks, vaso-vagal syncope is the classical example of very rapid, simultaneous or parallel activation of the SNS and the PNS [262]. In migraine pathophysiology, a large body of clinical and pharmacotherapeutic evidences indicates that intrinsic brain noradrenergic hyperfunction is not pathogenetic but rather protective. There appears to be sufficient evidence-based grounds to reconsider theories that presume a CNS or brain neuronal origin for migraine. A 'swing' in systemic or peripheral SNS function appears to develop between the attack-free phase (basal state hypofunction) and the pre-attack and attack phases (pain/arousal related hyperfunction, also see Chapter 8). The primary cranial physiological system involved in migraine must be afforded a striking but limited degree of 'protection' by systemic / peripheral SNS hypofunction (headache-free periods) as well as by a diffuse peripheral and brain neuronal autonomic (SNS and PNS) activation (during migraine attacks).

Although no amount of supportive evidence ever proves a case, a hypothesis may be refuted by a single piece of contradictory evidence. – K.R. Popper.

Chapter 6

PUPIL, EYELID, AND MIGRAINE

Conventionally, pupillary size is believed to be determined by a functional mutually-antagonistic balance between autonomically innervated constrictor and dilator muscle fibres of the iris sphincter. As a readily accessible non-invasive 'window' to the brain and the ANS, study of the pupil and associated eye signs has evoked much interest in migraine research as well as in other diverse fields. Investigation of pupillary dysfunction might offer some insight into the elusive pathophysiological basis of migrainous headache. The present overall consensus opinion is that during the headache-free period in migraine patients a deficiency of sympathetic terminal NE stores within the pupil prevails and is associated with a postsynaptic adrenergic receptor hypersensitivity [31,263]. That such pupillary constriction represents a 'mild' paralytic Horner syndrome in 5%-20% of migraine patients in the headache-free periods [31,264,265] as well as during headache attacks [31,264-267], however, appears debatable. The mechanistic basis for development of 'mild' or 'partial' Horner syndrome in migraine or cluster headache remains uncertain.

Almost fifty years ago, Walsh and O'Doherty suggested that swelling of the internal carotid artery (ICA) during migraine attacks could cause ophthalmoplegia either by direct compression or ischemia of the involved nerves; narrowing of the ICA was seen in two of three selected cases [268]. Pupillary miosis in migraine is believed to result from a cervical sympathetic deficiency from such a compressive-ischemic process involving the ICA [264-269]. Despite general availability of advanced neuroimaging techniques over last two decades, however, ICA swelling / narrowing has not again been seen in migraine patients. Also, miosis has not been associated with migraine-like symptoms including scintillating scotomata following ICA dissection [270-273]. Third, miosis in primary vascular headaches is bilateral and the smaller pupil is not necessarily on the side of the headache in patients with usually unilateral headache indicating a non-lateralizing cranial autonomic phenomenon [264-266,269] rather than a lateralizing neurological deficit. Fourth, miosis is not specific to migraine attacks, with anisocoria having been recorded in headache-free intervals in 'non-specific' headache attacks, cluster headache, episodic tension-type headache, and muscle contraction headache (tension-type headache) [264,274-276]. Conversely, mydriasis has been associated with migraine attacks [277-285]. *Finally, swelling and contrast enhancement of the affected nerve that resolves spontaneously or after steroid treatment has been reported on MRI in most but not all patients with ophthalmoplegic migraine (OM) [286-290] shifting the pathogenetic focus for OM from the ICA to the cranial nerve-brainstem junction.* The limitations of the compressive, ischemic, and demyelinating hyptheses for OM have been discussed [291,292]. The postulated pathogenetic role for ICA swelling in the genesis of OM or miosis (in headache-free intervals or during migraine attacks) appears untenable. Also, interruption of parasympathetic innervation – postganglionic parasympathetic paresis (Adie's tonic pupil) -- rather than sympathetic overactivity might underlie transient or more prolonged (? persistent) mydriasis accompanying migraine [279,283,293,294], although it remains uncertain how such a peripheral, unilateral neuroparalytic parasympathetic defect might develop during migraine attacks. Neuropeptide-mediated antidromic inflammation of ocular parasympathetic fibres (short ciliary nerves) in neuro-anatomical proximity with the nasociliary branch of V 1 fibres at the ciliary ganglion is one plausible explanation (see further).

In the context of current understanding of migraine pathogenesis, pupillary aberrations (both miosis and mydriasis) during and inbetween attacks, thus, remain inexplicable. Nine issues merit careful analysis: (i) *Contrary to older concepts, the two limbs of the ANS – sympathetic and parasympathetic -- are not really antagonistic* [33,37,224,225,262,295, see Chapter 5]. ***The pupil is a classic example of synchronized activity of the two limbs of the ANS, although the synchrony is currently misunderstood.*** Although darkness or arousal-related (psycho-sensory) mydriasis is commonly regarded primarily as a sympathetically mediated reflex [31], partial pupillary dilatation in darkness in the human sympathectomized eye does occur; on the other hand, a well-defined degree of central sympathetic tone is necessary for full development of miosis [33,105,296,297]. Importantly, the miosis of Horner's syndrome is never maximal and is usually slight [298]. (ii) The psycho-sensory restitution phenomenon -- pupillary constriction to light after induced fatigue -- is maintained after sympathectomy of the II and the III neurons but is abolished or diminished by a hypothalamic lesion affecting the I sympathetic neuron, a lesion in the III (oculomotor) nucleus or in the connecting pathways between the sympathetic and the III nucleus [298]. This miotic reflex is, thus, a central sympathetic reflex affecting the control of the sympathetic center over the constrictor center [298]. (iii) In migraine and cluster headache patients with eyes signs, miosis and ptosis frequently do not manifest in parallel. Over thirty years ago, a subtle dissociation between ptosis and miosis was seen during attacks in cluster headache [299]. More recently, in migraine patients with unilateral headache [265-267] and cluster headache patients [274], on average, eyelid separation was greater on the symptomatic side, unequivocally suggesting ipsilateral greater sympathetic activity [296,297]. Less consistent development of ptosis along with miosis during attacks and greater recovery than miosis during headache-free intervals in both migraine [266] and in cluster headache [267] patients stimulated the *speculation* that pupillary sympathetic fibres are more vulnerable than or separate from those sympathetic fibres destined for the eyelid within the internal carotid plexus [2666,299]. *The other more logical explanation is that pain- and arousal-related SNS activity increases during painful attacks of migraine as well as cluster headache possibly through activation of the locus ceruleus in the brainstem [300], and, in conjunction with attack-related parasympathetic activation effects both miosis and eyelid retraction on the symptomatic side* [224,225,296,297]. In patients with frequent severe migraine attacks attending tertiary care headache centers, the headache-free periods are unlikely to be free from a basal state of ANS activation due to residual arousal (discussed later, section 8) that might contribute to miosis between attacks. (iv) Electrical stimulation of the infratrochlear nerve causes transient ipsilateral decrease in pupil area by 20% in normal volunteers for 3-4 minutes; antidromic discharge in the trigeminal nerve is likely involved [301]. In contrast, mechanical stimulation of the trigeminal nerve, both with and without stellate ganglionectomy, was found to be highly effective in causing intense intraocular vasodilatation, rise of IOP, and pupillary miosis; similar to electrical stimulation [301], an axon (antidromic) reflex is probably involved [105]. The theoretical basis for occurrence of episodic prodromal and 'pre-prodromal' IOP rises in migraine has been elucidated [19,107,302,303]. Asymmetry of IOP with significantly (~50%) higher value on the side ipsilateral to the migraine headache has been reported in a single patient [293]. A mechanical neuropeptide-linked IOP-rise related component for the miosis observed in migraine patients cannot be excluded. (v) The serotonergic system (peripheral or central / brain or both) exerts an important role in determining the state of the pupil. Mianserin, a tetracyclic antidepressant and a clinically effective drug for migraine prevention [304], induces a dose-related reduction of the pupillary diameter in healthy volunteers [305,306] and constricted pinpoint pupils unresponsive to naloxone or dilated pupils in patients with overdose [307]. ICI 169,369 and ICI 170,809 are other 5-HT$_2$ receptor antagonists that induce dose-related miosis in volunteers [319,310]. Buspirone, a partial agonist for 5-HT$_{1A}$ receptors, also causes dose-dependent miosis in humans [311]. Although in terms of its anti-migraine action and on the basis of in vitro 5-HT receptor affinity, mianserin has been grouped with other potent 5-HT$_2$ receptor blockers (methysergide, pizotifen, cyproheptadine) [304], antidepressants (tricyclic or tetracyclic) can cause the serotonin syndrome [312; also see section 9] while cyproheptadine -- an established and functional 5-HT$_2$ receptor blocker -- can rapidly reverse the marked mydriasis seen in this condition [313]. Mydriasis seen in serotonin syndrome is consistent with the ability of serotonin and serotonomimetic agents like fenfluramine or indalpine to effect pupillary dilatation [314-316]. (vi) A subtle subclinical **cortical-level** control on the pupil is also suggested by development of episodic miosis (as frequently as five times per hour) with loss of the light reflex but without change in lid position in a patient with partial seizures; the attacks were associated with EEG discharges of the left temporo-occipital region [317]. Conversely, generalized tonic-clonic [318] or hysterical [319] seizures are often associated with bilateral mydriasis due to central sympathetic overactivity. As reviewed, in animals, electrical stimulation of different cortical regions can result in pupillary constriction or dilatation [317]. (vii) Non-muscarinic miosis is a component of the ocular irritative response in man as well as in animals; cholecystokinin, C-terminal fragments of CGRP, and AVP are neuropeptides possibly involved [320]. (viii) Bilateral alterations of pupil function, both mydriasis as well as miosis (without changes in lid position), have been found in disorders associated with variable degrees of ANS hypofunction including amyloidosis, pure autonomic failure, diabetes and other less common conditions while unilateral Horner-like miosis (without ptosis) was detected in multiple system atrophy [321]. Such non-lateralizing pupillary changes are difficult to rationalize in the conceptual mould of neuroparalytic syndromes such as Holmes-Adie or Horner's syndrome and likely represent a non-paralytic outcome of multiple influences at the level of the brain and the eye [322]. Two, hypersensitivity to dilute tropicamide (0.01%) in early Alzheimer's disease or progressive supranuclear palsy [323,324], combined hypersensitivity to both epinephrine as well as to methacholine in Hashimoto's thyroiditis [325], and progressive increase in pupil cycle time in chronic alcoholism [326] might also be rationalized in the context of combined influences of cognition-arousal related brain activation and local ocular influences on pupillary function [322]. (ix) Enhanced ciliospinal reflex in attack-free cluster headache patients in the absence of denervation hypersensitivity points to a state of sympathetic pre-ganglionic hyperfunction [327] while bilateral enhanced pupillary mydrisasis to tyramine but not to phenylepinephrine in cluster headache patients in prolonged remission excludes 'denervation effect' but indicates an enhanced ability to release NE from the pre-synaptic (post-ganglionic) sympathetic nerve endings [328].

In summary, pupillary changes in migraine, whether noted during the headache-free periods or during headache probably reflect the outcome of a complex interaction between local ocular (neuropeptide, ANS influences, and mechanical IOP-related) and higher hypothalamic / cortical neuronal activation. A functional synergism prevails naturally between the SNS and the PNS at the level of the pupil; during clinical pupillary testing, this physiological synergism is routinely overcome pharmacologically by sympathomimetic mydriatics and parasympathomimetic miotics. Fundamentally, heightened central ANS (sympathetic and parasympathetic) tone will generally reduce pupil size and reactions to light including maximum constriction velocity. Uncommonly in life (generalized tonic-clonic seizures or hysterical seizures or panic/anxiety neurosis disorder) or as a pre-agonal / agonal phenomenon, active central suppression of pupillary miotic influence will lead to stress-related mydriasis. Pupillary miosis in vascular headaches is usually bilateral. In the context of non-paralytic bilateral alterations in pupil function, the role of clinical pharmacological evaluation for pupillary denervation hypersensitivity is confusing and can be misleading. There is no technique to eliminate the central autonomic / serotonergic / non-muscarinic effects of arousal (that can last for several days after a migraine attack) on peripheral laboratory measures of pupillary function. The pupil is not the specific biological disease 'marker' actively sought by researchers in diverse fields [322]. *Extrapolating about disease mechanisms in primary vascular headaches from simplistic laboratory observations of the pupil size will increase -- not decrease -- the extant pathophysiological confusion.*

There was not the non-existent nor the existent then ;
There was not the air nor the heaven which is beyond.
What did it contain? Where? In whose protection?
Was there water, unfathomable, profound?...

From Vedic 'Hymn of Creation' (c. 1400 BC)

Table 3. Nature of migrainous clinical and laboratory phenomena

Feature/Phenomenon	Adaptive phenomena	Epiphenomena	Pathogenetic
Nausea / vomiting	++ (AVP)		
Facial Pallor ; Raynaud's phenomenon	+ (AVP)		
Fluid retention	+ (AVP)		
Facial / Ocular congestion; Sweating		++	
Dizziness / Vertigo		++	
Hypotension / Orthostatic features	++		
Ocular hypotony	+		
Photophobia		+	
Lacrimation		+	
Sonophobia		+	
Osmophobia		+	
Episodic daytime sleepiness	++ (AVP)		
Tinnitus		++	
Yawning	++ (AVP)		
Pupillary Aberrations		+ +	
Parasympathetic activation: peripheral features (gastric stasis, prolonged PR-interval)	+	+/-	
Parasympathetic activation: central antinociception	+		
Evoked potentials / Event-related slow potentials; Habituation deficit	+		
Platelet aggregation	+/-		
Platelet MAO-inhibitor activity ↓	+/-		
Antiphospholipid antibodies	+/-	+	
Magnesium depletion in plasma (hypomagnesemia) and brain	++		
Cutaneous allodynia	+/-	+/-	
Prolactin ↑	++	+/-	
Cortisol ↑	+		
Vasopressin (AVP) ↑	++		

Plasma norepinephrine release; brain noradrenergic activation	+		
Plasma serotonin ↑	++		
Brain serotonergic activation	++		
Dopaminergic hyperactivity	+		
Melatonin	+ (?AVP)		
Patent Foramen Ovale	++		

Key: AVP – Arginine Vasopressin; ++ Probable / Likely; + Possible; +/- Uncertain / Indeterminate; ↑-- increase ; ↓ -- decrease.

Chapter 7

PROLACTIN, MELATONIN, STRESS, AND MIGRAINE

A complex and uncertain relation prevails between aberrations of prolactin, melatonin, and migraine. Alterations in prolactin and melatonin secretion suggest a hypothalamic chronobiologic involvement in migraine; however, the cause/effect debate has not been resolved.

Migraine seems likely to occur when prolactin secretion is elevated, e.g., with stress, oversleeping, premenstrual period, or estrogen or oral contraceptive therapy [329]. Administration of sodium valproate, a proven category migraine preventive agent [2], however, does not influence prolactin secretion in migraine patients [330]. Two, flunarizine, a calcium antagonist used for migraine prophylaxis [249], unexpectedly, worsens the migraine index significantly in non-responders [331]. Remarkably, acute and chronic administration of flunarizine to healthy women and female migraine patients, respectively, *increases* prolactin secretion [332]. Three, whereas bromocriptine lowers systemic blood pressure in migraine patients as well as IOP in normal volunteers (discussed previously) and lowers prolactin hypersecretion, ***hyperprolactinemia is known to increase the IOP*** [333]. To a certain degree, an inverse relation prevails between ocular choroidal blood flow and IOP; a higher basal IOP can dampen sudden rises of choroidal blood flow [19,200]. ***Strikingly, most states with pronounced hyperprolactinemia, including prolactinomas, are not associated with migraine.*** Also, prolactin concentrations rise during sleep, while sleep commonly relieves an ongoing migraine attack (see Chapter 3). Nevertheless, in migraine pathophysiology, it is prudent not to overemphasize the clinical significance of the effect of prolactin itself on IOP. Four, oral or intravenous administration of 10 mg of metoclopramide to adult men raises serum prolactin concentrations by approximately 6-fold for up to 9 and 2 hours, respectively [334]. Metoclopramide is finding use as a migraine attack-aborting agent; relatively large doses upto 80 mg have been administered intravenously [100,101]. The prominent effect of metoclopramide on prolactin secretion, however, does not support a migraine pathogenetic role for the latter. Five, while baseline prolactin levels are generally normal in migraine patients, a hyper-responsive prolactin release following administration of thyrotropin releasing hormone has been shown during migraine attacks [335]. Also, a decreased nocturnal prolactin peak but with higher cortisol levels has been shown in patients with chronic migraine [336]. Plasma cortisol concentrations significantly increase during acute migraine attacks and migraine intensity correlated with plasma cortisol elevations.[1] Corticosteroids have been used as treatment for severe migraine attacks, in the treatment of sustained or status migraine, in the treatment of drug-overuse headache (oral or intravenous corticosteroids), and in the treatment of immunosuppressant-induced headache in organ transplant recipients.[2] The use of corticosteroids in these clinical circumstances is empiric and the outcome is not always predictable. Besides, prolonged migraine states can spontaneously subside unpredictably. Nevertheless, a cranial vascular 'stabilization' effect cannot be excluded. Also, acute increases (within hours) have been reported following corticosteroid administration in primary open angle glaucoma (POAG). *About 5% of the general population will have a change in intraocular pressure of greater than 15 mm Hg when challenged with corticosteroids while approximately 90% of patients with POAG will have a raised intraocular pressure when challenged with corticosteroids.*[3] Decreased aqueous humour outflow facility at the trebecular meshwork probably underlies the ocular hypertensive effect of corticosteroids. High-dose corticosteroid therapy can raise the IOP in responsive migrane patients, that in concert with the anti-inflammatory cranial vascular 'stabilization' effect, may dampen choroidal blood flow and abort the attack. Six, metoclopramide – a fairly established migraine aborting pharmacologic agent -- stimulates prolactin release, with the peak response being greater following oral rather than i.v. administration.[4] Seven, stress-related prolactin release counters many of the immunosuppressive effects of corticosteroids [337].

Increased readiness of the prolactin-release promoting system during migraine attacks is best viewed as an anticipatory/event-related adaptive response

---

[1] G. Juhasz et al. Headache 2007; 47:371-383.

[2] T.D. Rozen. Current Treatment Options in Neurology 2002;4:395-401.

[3] Bernal et al. Lancet 2000;355:577.

[4] K. Ijaiya. European Journal of Pediatrics 1980;134:231-237.

to stress [37]. The neuro-physiology of sleep itself is complex and incompletely understood; myriad factors can influence nocturnal prolactin levels. As discussed previously (Chapter 5), clinical features that indicate attack-related dopaminergic hyperactivity / hypersensitivity must not be construed to reflect pathogenetic phenomena. Dopaminergic hyperactivity is fundamentally associated with lower prolactin levels. Prolactin does not appear to be directly involved in migraine pathogenesis. Conversely, high IOP in states of hyperprolactinemia may limit ocular choroidal flow and keep migraine in remission.

In striking contrast to hyperprolactinemia, melatonin lowers IOP in man [338]. Melatonin synthesis is acutely suppressed in humans by exposure to sunlight and artificial light (2500 lux) but not light of ordinary indoor intensity [339]. Aretaeus (A.D. 81-?) noted the tendency of migraine patients to shun light: "…they flee the light; the darkness soothes their disease; nor can they bear to look upon (or hear) anything disagreeable…" [45]. The artist Coleman's retreat to the darkroom, insurance woes, and isolation due to frequent migraine attacks spurred his creativity towards unique use of alternative process photography [http://www.migraines.org/about/abouawar.htm]. Also, The Migraine Trust recommends polychromatic dark glasses for cutting down glare [http://www.migrainetrust.org/C2B/ document_tree/ViewADocument.asp?ID=26andCatID=24]; the efficacy of this measure in preventing migraine attacks, however, remains uncertain. High-intensity light suppression of melatonin may, in part, explain the photosensitivity / photophobia of most migraine patients. Lower plasma values of melatonin following exposure to high-intensity light [339], in female migraine patients [340], and chronic migraine patients with insomnia [336], can permit episodic rises in IOP and increase the susceptibility of patients to develop migraine attacks. Melatonin can, however, itself precipitate headache in migraine patients.[5] *Lowering of IOP without directly limiting choroidal blood flow is the most likely pathophysiological mechanism involved in precipitation of such drug-induced headaches.*

The IOP is one system on which prolactin and melatonin exert opposite, mutually-antagonistic, possibly balancing influences; however, the IOP is overall affected by a very large number of internal homeostatic and external influences. Besides, the sedative effect of melatonin was observed at the time of its initial description [341] and was confirmed subsequently by administration in the evening [342]. Further, in an open study, melatonin was shown to prevent occurrence of migraine attacks.[343] Finally, the pineal gland exerts an inhibitory

---

[5] Unpublished personal observation.

impact on both vaspressin biosynthesis and secretion; while endogenous melatonin mediates these effects, exogenously administered melatonin does not modify neurohypophysial AVP content or AVP release in pinealectomized male rats or in Syrian hamster exposed to light for long periods or challenged with hyperosmotic solutions [344,345]. Melatonin inhibits spontaneous neuronal activity in the suprachiasmatic nucleus, an effect consistent with inhibition by melatonin of spontaneous (and vasoactive intestinal peptide-induced) increase and accelerated decrease of AVP release in dispersed cells of the rat suprachiasmatic nucleus [346]. Remarkably, exposure to short photoperiod for 4 or 10 weeks increased vasopressin content in the hamster pituitary neurointermediate lobe. [345] Avoidance behavior is a typical feature of migraine patients, including aversion to bright lights, suspected foods and alcoholic beverages, and sexual intercourse.[13,46,170] The pineal gland and its hormone, melatonin, may interact with the vasopressin-oxytocin system to define avoidance behavior.[347] Ophthalmic (elevated IOP and large cup-to-disk ratios) and illumination factors might have an additive effect on the timing of melatonin excretion, which in turn might predispose individuals to experience early morning awakenings.[348,349] Interestingly, some migraine patients regularly wake up from sleep early with migraine headache; such headaches are more frequently associated with REM sleep .[170,186]

In summary, as part of the complex neuro-endocrine activation that develops in migraine, aberrations of prolactin and melatonin release might define the susceptibility but do not appear to be central to the pathogenesis of the disorder. Despite the species differences, experimental circadian neuroendocrine features related to melatonin release could have relevance to migraine pathophysiology. AVP secretion or suppression and its possible link to IOP homeostasis appears to be the final common pathway involved in the influence of both prolactin and melatonin on occurence of migraine attacks. Response of AVP release to sunlight or hight intensity artificial light has not yet been studied in humans, but might have a direct bearing on the characteristic aversion of migraine patients to bright light.

The desire for results that would confirm our beliefs drives us to subvert randomised controlled trials.—C. Martyn. Lancet 1996;347:70.

Chapter 8

EVOKED POTENTIALS, MIGRAINE, AND AROUSAL

Obviously, science follows no plan. It develops at random…Men of science do not know where they are going. They are guided by chance, by subtle reasoning, by a sort of clairvoyance. – Alexis Carrel.

Lack of habituation or even potentiation of evoked and event-related cortical potentials during repetition of the same stimuli is regarded as the best reproducible inter-ictal (between attacks) electrophysiological abnormality in MA+ and MA- patients [350,351]. The habituation 'deficit' appears to be involved also in studies of somatosensory evoked potentials [351], auditory-evoked cortical responses [352] and visually-evoked potentials [353] in migraine patients between attacks. While the cause, course, biological role or nature, and consistency of the habituation 'deficit' remains uncertain [20,350,354,355,356], increased contingent negative variation (CNV) amplitude -- a specific noradrenergic activity-dependent event-related slow potential -- between attacks in migraine patients is believed to offer convincing support to the biobehavioral model of migraine [17,18]. CNV, that undoubtedly reflects CNS activity [357,358], has, however, been found aberrant more commonly in MA- patients than in MA+ patients [359], a profile which is quite the *reverse* of what might be expected generally as well as in the context of the biobehavioral model of migraine. Finally, hypersensitivity to light or noise is a migraine attack-related phenomenon; nevertheless, such hypersensitivity cannot be used to support the concept of cerebral cortex hyperexcitability between attacks.***Overall, contradictory laboratory evidences for both increased and decreased cortical excitability as well as decreased and normal function of inhibitory cortical*** *inter-neurones are available; there is no definitive knowledge about neural generators involved in high frequency oscillations* [20,350].

A clearer conceptual distinction is required regarding the state of brain physiology in migraine patients between the headache phase and the headache-free phase.[20] While aura / headache-pain related brain neuronal arousal during migraine attacks cannot be argued, the state of brain neuronal activity (hypoactive, hyperactive, or normal) as well as its biological role during headache-free intervals is pathophysiologically important but rather vague. The key issue involved is whether migraine patients are stress- or arousal-free during the headache-free intervals. *Several features suggest that migraine patients with frequent attacks (say, one or more every week) maintain a variable, unpredictable, possibly continuous but subclinical state of stress that can alter responses to evoked potentials even in the absence of painful attacks of headache (with or without aura)*: (i) As discussed previously (Chapter 5), the prodrome of migraine can extend to several hours or days during which time-interval initiation of the attack has begun, and, patients can no longer be regarded as being in the basal non-stressed physiological state; (ii) MA+ or MA- attacks are associated with substantial increases in plasma methionine-enkephalin, which return to baseline only slowly (over weeks) in the pain-free period.[360] (iii) Migraine attack-related inconsistently lateralized prolonged cranial vasodilatation persists for 48 hours after cessation of headache, subsiding gradually to normal levels by six days.[361] Such protracted cranial vasodilatation would expectedly be accompanied by a significant level of residual arousal / brain activation. (iv) Occurrence of stress below the threshold of headache attacks is distinctly possible in migraine patients.[362] Since evoked potentials in migraine basically study stress-associated arousal accompanying perceptions of challenge, threat, harm/loss, and coping options (primary and secondary appraisals),[363] consideration of operation of a continuum of stress-related arousal and altered evoked potentials is plausible and useful.[20] *Based on entirely subjective perception of pain, functional personal and economic disability, and socio-professional embarrassment tantamount to a stigma,*[363,364] *arousal responses vary from migraine patient to patient and even in the same patient on different occasions; reproducibility of evoked responses in the same or different cohort is, therefore, likely to be practically impossible.*[20] (v) Propranolol – through ß-blockade -- cannot be expected to improve [20] the putatively reduced noradrenergic-dependent thalamo-cortical excitation between headache attacks. [350] (vi) The migraine preventive role of amitriptyline and of the combination of amitriptyline and propranolol – with opposite influences on brain neuronal functions -- also challenges the proposed role of 'defective habituation' in the pathogenesis of migraine.[20] *Propranolol and amitriptyline have opposite effects on bioavailability of AVP, decreasing and increasing the release of anti-diuretic hormone, respectively. The synergistic effect for migraine prevention of this otherwise illogical combination very likely depends upon a combination of peripheral ocular effects and CNS release of AVP.*

Overall, more often than not, the early phases of arousal in migraine patients keep both the aura as well as the headache at bay.[19,20,22,36,37] Post-stress headache is a characteristic feature of migraine and electrophysiological responses in the early continuum, regardless of the precise source of generation, are probably reflective of physiological adaptation involving a learned conservation of neuronal functional 'potential' or 'energy' for a more demanding attack-related challenge that generally follows subsequently.[20,36] Conceptually, the 'protective' or 'adaptive' role of the early phase of brain arousal in migraine patients helps to maintain a broad neuro-physiological perspective. That such physiological alterations support the biobehavioral model of migraine is a highly contentious issue that falls well into the category of speculation. All formulatons of the role of the monoaminergic system in migraine, including the biobehavioral model are indirect and inferential. To dismiss a formulation about migraine mechanisms due to lack of proper scientific backing[1], stimulates the question: *"What indeed is proper scientific backing in migraine"* ? *What masquerades as 'proper' science in migraine is a huge catalogue of myths and speculations; what is even worse is that these conjectures are completely disconnected from each other.* Even if, in the remote future, we might be able to directly study brain monoaminergic function in migraine, such study would have to done for protracted periods in the pre-prodromal phase – a truly formidable if not impossible research enterprise.

Table 4. BBB Penetrability and Migraine Pharmacology

	(Intact) BBB penetration	CNS Effects relevant to Migraine Pathophysiology
Alcohol	++	↓ Release of AVP
Nicotine [71,236,237]	++	↑ Release of AVP, β-endorphin, ACH, NE, Dopamine, 5-HT, ACTH
Reserpine	++	↓ reuptake of brain NE and 5-HT; does not precipitate migraine aura / scintillating scotoma

1 A. Fumal et al. Brain, July 2006; 129: E53.

Table 4. (Continued)

	(Intact) BBB penetration	CNS Effects relevant to Migraine Pathophysiology
Magnesium [160-164]	+/-	No known neuronal effect; experimentally, attenuates BBB permeability; basis of anti- convulsive action in eclampsia uncertain
Serotonin (Plasma)	-	-
Norepinephrine (Plasma)	-	-
Arginine-vasopressin (Plasma) [374,375]	+	Antinociception and behavior control [37]
Botulinum toxin	-	No genuine antinociceptive effect in the absence of skeletal muscle spasm [180]
Lisinopril [366,367,368]	+/-	No definitive brain neuronal effect
Candesartan cilexetil [369]	+/-	No definitive brain neuronal effect
Riboflavine [372,373]	-	No definitive brain neuronal effect
Propranolol	++	β-blockade (central & peripheral), brain 5-HT antagonism
Metoprolol	+/-	β-blockade (peripheral)-hydrophilic
Atenolol [209,240,241]	-	β-blockade (peripheral)-hydrophilic
Timolol [370,371]	-	β-blockade (peripheral)-hydrophilic
Nadolol [209]	-	β-blockade (peripheral)-hydrophilic
Verapamil [249]	-	No definitive brain neuronal effect
Nifedipine [249]	-	No definitive brain neuronal activity, yet aborts migraine aura

Drug		Notes
Flunarizine [249]	++	↑ Prolactin; ↓ BBB permeability in acute experimental hypertension [379]
Nitroglycerin (NO donor) [380]	++	Alters brain monoamines; no definitive brain neuronal effect; NO ↑ BBB permeability in rats [381-383]; nitroglycerin *aborts* migraine aura but *precipitates* migraine headache
m-CPP	++	5-HT$_{2A}$ receptor antagonist, 5-HT$_{2C}$ receptor agonist; precipitates migraine-like headaches
Amitriptyline	++	Noradrenergic and serotonergic agonist; ↑ AVP release
Mianserin	++	Noradrenergic and serotonergic agonist
Caffeine	++	Noradrenergic stimulant
Cocaine	++	Noradrenergic, serotonergic, dopaminergic stimulant
Amphetamine	++	Noradrenergic stimulant
Fluoxetine (SSRI)	++	Serotonergic stimulant
Venlafaxine [376]	++	Selective noradrenergic and serotonergic agonist
Phenelzine [377]	++	Adrenergic agonist
Phenelzine and atenolol [377]		Combination efficacy inexplicable [20]
Propranolol and amitriptyline [378]	++	Combination efficacy inexplicable [144]
Cyproheptadine	++	Serotonergic antagonist
Methysergide	++	Serotonergic antagonist
Pizotifen [365]	++	Serotonergic antagonist
Sodium valproate	++	? Cortical 'stabilization' [251,384]; analgesic [385,386]

Table 4. (Continued)

	(Intact) BBB penetration	CNS Effects relevant to Migraine Pathophysiology
Topiramate	++	? Cortical 'stabilization' [251,384]; analgesic [385]
Gabapentin	++	? Cortical 'stabilization' [251,384]; analgesic [385]
Donepezil	++	PNS (peripheral and central) agonist; analgesic
Apomorphine	++	Dopamine agonist
Metoclopramide	++	Dopamine antagonist
Estrogen [387]	++	↑ AVP bioavailability [37]; restores postmenopausal lost inhibitory opoid tonus [92]
Aspirin	++	Peripheral and central analgesic actions [388]
NSAIDs	++	Peripheral and central analgesic actions [388]

Key: ++ free / ready crossing of intact BBB; +/- limited/uncertain crossing of intact BBB; - poor/negligible crossing of intact BBB; ? - uncertain mechanisms; ACH – acetylcholine; SSRI – selective serotonin reuptake inhibitor; NSAIDs – Non-steroidal anti-inflammatory drugs.

In summary, study of evoked potentials in migraine constitutes an interesting physiological phenomenon that is *unexpectedly* seen more often in MA- patients, presents formidable logistic challenge for replication, and, cannot, however, be integrated into a defensible overarching pathogenetic theory for migraine.The biological purpose or nature of this phenomenon remains elusive but cannot be dissociated from the arousal of recurrent painful migraine attacks. In patients with frequent migraine attacks, the headache-free cannot be regarded as a stress-free or baseline physiological state. *If both brain noradrenergic suppression (induced by propranolol) and excitation (induced by amitriptyline) can prevent migraine, a reorganization of concepts is essential.*

Research is rarely an activity free of ideological roots. There is no such thing as "purely objective" observation. -- P. Medawar.

Chapter 9

THE PLATELET-SEROTONIN-BRAIN NEURONAL CONNECTION: MILESTONE OR MILLSTONE?

The dangers of "falling in love with your hypothesis" and letting your "expectations shape your findings" are common pitfalls for the enthusiastic researcher. – Editorial. Lancet 1993;364:468.

Serotonin (5-hydroxytryptamine) was discovered in 1954 by Irvine Page [389]. While the first known action of 5-HT was that of a powerful vasoconstrictor, it is now known to be an important neurotransmitter in the brain [390] as well as a vasodilator (discussed further). On the basis of substantial but *indirect or circumstantial* evidence,[390] 5-HT stands implicated in migraine pathogenesis since ~50 years.[304,391-393] Free (circulating) 5-HT, that does not cross the BBB, is believed to sensitize the cranial arterial wall to pain.[393,394] (table 4). Nothwithstanding the virtual *absence* in platelets of the 5-HT synthesizing enzyme, tryptophan hydroxylase, the platelet is *believed* to be an excellent peripheral model that mirrors pre- and post-synaptic functions of the CNS serotonergic neurons [395-397]. Data linking alterations in 5-HT in body fluids (platelet, plasma, urine, and cerebrospinal fluid) are fragmentary and often conflicting; changes in platelet 5-HT are neither specific nor causally related to migraine.[398]

A vague incompletely defined 5-HT-related metabolic disturbance prevails in migraine with ictal release of 5-HT from platelets occurring only in MA- patients [399]; since most patients (70%) might suffer both MA- or MA+ attacks on different occasions [400,401], it is difficult to rationalize such disparate findings between the major migraine variants as reflecting definitive trait or state features.

Although studies using *in vitro* models have contributed enormously in characterizing 5-HT receptors in cranial blood vessels and in studying the effects of several putative anti-migraine agents including the triptans, [393,398] there is no definitive evidence for pathogenetic involvement of the brain serotonergic system in migraine. [390] Neurotransmitters are secretory or excretory products of neurons; neurotransmitters can modulate neuronal function but cannot be regarded as substitutes for (or initiators of) neuronal function.[13] While a causal contribution to migraine pathophysiological events does not necessarily mean an "initiating" or "exclusive" role, currently direct knowledge of intrinsic brain serotonergic neuronal function is incomplete and rudimentary. Conversely, the migraine preventive effect of some 5-HT_2 receptor antagonists, such as methysergide and pizotifen, has reinforced the belief that brain serotonergic hyperfunction makes a significant contribution to migraine pathogenesis.[304] *Intrinsic brain neuronal 5-HT release is believed to be a key step in the genesis of CSD.*[18] The efficacy of 5-HT-agonists such as sumatriptan and other triptans (activating 5-HT receptors --'5-HT_1-like' receptors in the vasculature and 5-HT_{1D} receptors in nervous tissue [393]) in aborting acute attacks of migraine [304,394,398] has further stimulated such thinking amongst primary headache researchers. Such assumptions, nevertheless, have distorted certain pharmacological absolutes related to understanding of migraine.

A brief review of available evidences lends caution to the belief that brain intrinsic 5-HT activity or hyperfunction plays a substantial role in migraine pathogenesis. (i) No systemic influence, including the platelet-serotonin hypothesis can satisfactorily explain key clinical characteristics of migraine including onset and offset of migraine at different ages, lateralization and spread of headache from one side to the other, and post-stress headache [13,19-22,402]. (ii) While parenteral reserpine -- a NE- and 5-HT reuptake inhibitor that readily crosses the BBB -- may cause headache, typical migraine-attack associated features including aura / scintillating scotoma have never been reported to occur after reserpine administration.[85,86,390,403] (iii) Clinical or experimental states of excess 5-HT in humans ameliorate migraine headache or induce remission of migraine attacks.[390,403] Intravenous administration of 5-HT relieved the headache induced by reserpine as as well as spontaneous migraine attacks. [85,404] Also, development of carcinoid syndrome remarkably decreased migraine frequency and intensity leading to a complete remission with post-operative recurrence.[405] 5-HT excess in carcinoid syndrome induces, besides other aberrations, an episodic or sustained state of vasodilatation, reflected in the cutaneous flushing, telangiectases, and paroxysmal hypotension. 5-HT release is involved in basal nitric oxide (NO) release (besides shear stress as well as thrombin release from platelets); 5-HT-induced vasodilatation is impaired with hypercholesterolemia.[406,407] Vasodilatory capacity of 5-HT appears clinically relevant to migraine pathophysiology. Overall, vasodilation has, however, a complex role in migraine with the NO donor, nitroglycerin, paradoxically serving as both the best human model for migraine [148,393] as well as a well-known instantaneous migraine-aura aborting agent.[408] *Sustained* vasodilatation (steady release of 5-HT in carcinoid syndrome) with relatively low blood pressure (see Chapter 5, table 2) appears to keep migraine in remission while relatively *sudden* pharmacological vasodilatation (parenteral reserpine or nitroglycerin) precipitates migraine-like headache or migraine. Remarkably, while nitroglycerin can precipitate MA- [148,393], systemic vasodilatation has *never* been shown to induce MA+, including the scintillating scotoma – this facet of migraine pathophysiology has not been appropriately underscored. NO directly inhibits propagation of retinal spreading depression (RSD) in a concentration- and time-dependent manner; also, NO speeds up recovery of the intrinsic optical signal after the wavefront.[409] The direct role of 5-HT in RSD is currently unknown, but RSD might underlie the migrainous scintillating scotoma.[19] (iv) Evidence supporting migraine preventive effect of the anti-platelet agent aspirin is very limited. Reduction in attack frequency below 50% in only 3 of 28 patients in a double-blind cross-over study in doses far in excess (1500 mg daily) of the ideal anti-platelet dose indicates the poor therapeutic value of restricting platelet aggregation and peripheral 5-HT release in migraine.[410] (v) There is complete dissociation between drug effects on platelets of migraine patients on the one hand (aggregability, adenosine triphosphatase release, and thromboxane generation) and migraine symptoms on the other. Propranolol enhances platelet aggregability and thereby enhances peripheral 5-HT bioavailability in migraine patients.[411] Thromboxane A_2 (TxA_2) is a potent platelet aggregant; propranolol, atenolol, and metoprolol significantly raise measured plasma thromboxane B_2 levels (the stable metabolite of TxA_2).[411,412] Platelet hyperaggregability is found with high levels of stress in diverse medical conditions besides migraine, being accompanied by and presumably resulting from elevated circulating levels of catecholamines. Enhanced platelet activation following β-blocker therapy probably involves release of α_2-receptor mediated catecholamine effects following blockade of β_2-receptors.[411]. By itself, the platelet aggregating effect of β-blockers is a pharmacological *absolute* that virtually eliminates any possible pathogenetic role for 5-HT through platelet-release. (vi) Nicotine increases platelet aggregation, 5-HT [413] and thrombin [414] bioavailability but many (though, not all) migraine patients continue to smoke [69,415,416] possibly due to the antinociceptive action of nicotine as well the addictive nature (physical and/or

behavioral dependence) of smoking cigarettes.[70,71] (see Chapter 5; table 4)
(vii) A negative correlation exists between migraine and antibodies to
phospholipids (the membrane-binding moiety increasing platelet aggregability),
[417] suggesting that the presence of such antibodies confers a degree of
protection against development of migraine.[418] (viii) Migraine headache has
been reported in patients with thrombocytopenia.[419] (ix) Although platelet
aggregation and adhesion are commonly increased in diabetes mellitus, it is
hypogylcaemia rather than hyperglycaemia that precipitates migraine.[82,419] (x)
Menstrual migraine typically improves with pregnancy,[420] but estrogens
increase epinephrine-induced platelet aggregation.[421] (xi) Migraine-like
headache is a sequela of cocaine use,[173,174] but cocaine inhibits platelet
aggregation and dissociates preformed platelet aggregates.[422] (xii) Whereas
atherothrombotic disease and incidence of ischemic stroke with clear links to
platelet dysfunction generally advances with age, migraine generally remits with
advancing years.[13,46,423]. Also, ischaemic stroke is a rarity in younger
migraine subjects.[424]. The posterior cerebral artery is anatomically particularly
labile at its origin; rare occurrence of posterior cerebral circulation infarcts in the
migraine patient likely reflects the outcome of an idiosyncratic critical reduction
of perfusion in an anatomically vulnerable region.[171,418]. *Overall, there is but
little evidence to support the belief that serum / platelet serotonin function tells
us anything definite about brain neuronal function* [425]. *"...believing that
serum serotonin levels tell us anything about central (brain) serotonin is like
watching the sky in London to guess the weather in Sydney"* [426] – is an
analogy that is hard to improve upon. In any case, vasomotor activity resulting
from release of 5-HT in the periphery has been determined not to have significant
central cerebrovascular effect.[427]

   *The most important limitation of the serotonergic hypothesis for migraine is
the carefully structured pharmacological myth that several or most migraine
preventive drugs are serotonergic antagonists.* [304,428,429] A large variety of
actions are mediated by $5-HT_2$ receptors and several unrelated pharmacological
agents show $5-HT_2$ receptor antagonism.[304,429] Most antimigraine drugs,
including propranolol, amitriptyline, verapamil and nifedipine show *in vitro*
affinity to $5-HT_{1A}$ and/or $5-HT_2$ receptor subtypes in human brain; the affinity of
verapamil and nifedipine – *that do not readily cross the intact BBB* (table 4) -- for
the $5-HT_2$ receptor erroneously suggested that these calcium-channel blockers also
might exert a critical brain *in vivo* $5-HT_2$ receptor-antagonism.[429] Two
important but, unfortunately, false corollaries to this assumption have gathered
strength in the last few decades: (a) Serotonomimetic agents or agonists generally

induce or worsen migraine. (b) Migraine and depression are comorbid conditions with a shared pathogenesis or common pathogenetic pathways.

Critical limitations of such scientific thinking include the following: (i) While atenolol is currently regarded as a first-line migraine preventive agent, [241-246], it was found to be totally inactive *in vitro* at all three 5-HT receptor subtypes. [429] *Such key pharmacological findings that do not support current theories of migraine pathogenesis have simply been swept under the carpet, to be ignored and hopefully erased from the consciousness with passage of time.* Also, as discussed previously, atenolol does not readily cross the intact BBB and cannot possibly critically influence any brain neuronal function (table 4). (ii) Amitriptyline is an established migraine preventive agent.[2] Antidepressants increase synaptic 5-HT or NE or both and basically enhance monoaminergic neurotransmission at all levels of the CNS. There is overwhelming evidence form neuropharmacology and neuropsychiatry that amitriptyline (and other tricyclic or tetracyclic antidepressants like mianserin) is a *serotonomimetic* agent. *Induction of serotonin syndrome by amitriptyline and other antidepressants including selective serotonin reuptake inhibitors (SSRIs) in humans is the clearest clinical evidence for a brain 5-HT agonistic or serotonomimetic action of this group of drugs.*[312,430-433] The serotonin syndrome is thought to be induced by combined activation of the cAMP-related $5-HT_{1A}$ receptors and the phosphatidyl hydrolysis-linked $5-HT_2$ receptors.[312,432]. *Headache is neither included in the diagnostic criteria for nor commonly found in the serotonin syndrome.* [312,432] *Prevention of migraine by serotonomimetic agents is yet another pharmacological absolute (like BBB-related pharmacokinetic evidences related to atenolol, nadolol, or verapamil)* (table 4) *that has the potential to clear several myth-like assumptions linked to 5-HT and the pathogenesis of the disorder.* Till today, in migraine research there is no clear perception about the nature of alteration in brain serotonergic function by amitriptyline (or other tricyclic and tetracylic antidepressants). *There are several distinct references in the migraine literature about the 'anti-serotonergic' action of amitriptyline that completely ignore clinico-pharmacological reality; the NE and 5-HT re-uptake inhibitory action of amitriptyline has been, most unfortunately, equated with central / brain anti-serotonergic action by several migraine research groups. Even more unfortunately, no challenge has hitherto been mounted against this completely erroneous theoretical assumption.* (iii) Serotonin antagonists like cyproheptadine, pizotifen, and methysergide are also regarded as migraine preventive agents in the "proven" or well-accepted category".[2,304] However, methysergide, cyropheptadine, and propranolol can shorten the serotonin syndrome.[312,432]. *If pharmacologic drugs that have no possible action on brain serotonergic function (atenolol) or induce brain serotonergic hyperactivation (amitriptyline, mianserin, SSRIs, lithium, or imipramine) or effect brain serotonergic hypoactivation (methysergide, cyproheptadine, and propranolol) can all prevent migraine with approximately the same efficacy, it compels the consideration that brain serotonergic involvement is not the primary or key aberration in genesis of migraine.*[19-22,418,425,434] (iv) Neither the almost prototypical 5-HT$_2$ receptor blocker, ketanserin, [304,390] nor the the selective 5-HT$_2$ receptor antagonist ICI 169,369 [435] is effective in the prevention of migraine; 5-HT$_2$ receptor -- vascular or neuronal – activation, by itself, does not appear important in migraine pathogenesis. While ketanserin does not share the 5-HT$_{1C}$ binding property that pizotifen, cyproheptadine, methysergide, and mianserin possess,[304] the role of 5-HT$_{1C}$ receptors in migraine pathogenesis also remains uncertain. On the other hand, m-CPP, an experimental 5-HT$_{2A}$ receptor antagonist/5-HT$_{2A}$ receptor agonist, induces headaches in ~50% of both migraine patients and normal controls several hours after a single oral dose; notably, m-CPP does not release 5-HT from human platelets.[427,428] (v) *Unexpectedly, 5-HT$_2$ receptor antagonists tend to produce hyperalgesia.*[436] *Conversely, an overview of placebo-controlled RCTs offers unambiguous evidence for a powerful analgesic role of the serotonomimetic (and sympathomimetic) agent amitriptyline and other tricyclic antidepressants.* [437] Overall, combined brain serotonergic and adrenergic stimulation appears to have a positive influence on *antinociception* rather than a central role in migraine pathogenesis. (vi) While the promotion of cranial vasoconstriction by 5-HT$_2$ antagonists might contribute to prevention of migraine,[304] the instantaneous abolition of migraine aura with vasodilator drugs such as nitroglycerin, nifedipine, or isoproterenol [195,408] indicates that vascular changes are not central to the pathogenesis of migraine attacks. Also, while propranolol and other β-blockers are peripheral (including cranial) vasoconstrictors, verapamil and other calcium-channel antagonists are cranial vasodilators.[171] *This fact is not appreciated in migraine and cerebrovascular therapeutics but the difference in cerebral vasomotor activity between beta-blockers and calcium-channel antagonists can have important clinical consequences for individual patients, particularly those with primary vawcular headaches.* (vii) Use of propranolol is cautioned in patients with depression; however, common (but empiric) use of this agent to prevent migraine has not been associated with depression.[425] Besides, while reserpine can precipitate migraine-like headache (not aura) [85,405] and is linked to development of depression, the link between reserpine and depression itself is dubious and quite mythical.[438] *To avoid drawing fallacious conclusions from epidemiological associations, data regarding comorbidity must be knitted back* *into clinical evidences and the fundamentals of basic sciences.*[171] *Associations can be quite misleading: the close correlation between income-tax and lung cancer rates in the United States is a vivid example.*[439]

In summary, alterations in brain / central serotonergic function rather than platelet / peripheral function probably determine the tendency for migraine attacks to occur; however, such alterations are clearly secondary in nature. Brain serotonergic hyperfunction induced by pharmacologic agents (tricyclic or tetracyclic antidepressants or monoamine-oxidase inhibitors or SSRIs) tends to delay onset of migraine as well as to keep attacks in remission. *In vitro* affinity of 5-HT to 5-HT receptors types/subtypes in human or animal brain slices cannot be used to determine or predict clinically relevant *in vivo* pharmacological properties of anti-migraine drugs. Alterations in either density of 5-HT receptors/recptor subtypes or 5-HT levels in experimental animals following acute or prolonged exposures to antidepressants are very likely secondary or adaptive in nature; such findings must not be confused with primary clinically-relevant actions of serotonomimetic agents. Since drugs that do not possibly influence brain 5-HT function can prevent migraine, the site of origin of migraine remains unsettled. Conceptually, a balanced analysis of the serotonergic system does not support brain / brain-stem origin of migraine.

The resolution of a controversy entails bringing it onto the centre of the table, rather than sweeping it under the carpet. The components of a controversy must be re-read and re-examined dispassionately, a task ill-suited to those who have contributed to the structure of the controversy. Any controversy exists because extant scientific techniques cannot offer resolving data. At this juncture, logic generalization and extrapolation become paramount -- rather than further simplistic accretion of additional data – because they can address issues at the heart of the matter. At the centre of every controversy beats a heart of ignorance with a maddening undecipherable rhythm, a cosmic taunt to the so-called human intellect.

CONCLUSION

A profound conceptual confusion envelopes migraine theory and therapy. Drugs with strikingly opposite pharmacologic properties are commonly used empirically for preventing migraine, either alone or in combination. Closure of PFO or scalp injection of botulinum toxin are other purely empirical procedures. Such therapeutic endeavors and their underlying theoretical bases constitute a serendipitous and incoherent patchwork of mutually contradictory ideas struggling for dominance amongst migraine researchers. Little pathophysiological clarity is offered by either the vast phenomenology of migraine or by the elaborate system of classification of primary headaches. Several experimental migraine models, based on involvement of vascular or neuronal or trigeminovascular systems, are available; while *in vitro* models have characterized cranial blood vessel receptors and helped to study effects of putative anti-migraine agents, no model encompasses all vital facets of the disorder. The causal physiological aberration of migraine lies embedded in the 'pre-prodromal' and prodromal phases that are, in turn, less accessible or inaccessible to laboratory measures. Several first-line migraine preventive agents do not freely cross the intact BBB and challenge the presumed origin of the entity at the level of the brain. Also, significant delay in onset of migraine attacks indicates operation of adaptive stress-related physiological mechanisms, involving vasopressinergic, noradrenergic, and serotonergic systems that contribute to vasomotor control, antinociception, and behavior control. Such an adaptive system brings a semblance of order among the protean physiological disturbances observed in migraine and thereby bridges several seemingly unconnected or conflicting pathways of evidence. The mechanistic basis of migrainous headache and vomiting does not appear to be identical. A preliminary working template is suggested to separate adaptive, epiphenomenal, and pathogenetic mechanisms in migraine in the quest for the research vision for the entity.

Much work still remains to flesh out further the concept of adaptive mechanisms in migraine in order to integrate findings such as elevations of elastase (Tzourio et al., Ann. Neurol. 2000;47:648-651) and endothelin (Tzourio et al., Neurology 2001;56:1273-1277). Genetic associations / polymorphisms detected in migraine patients, including familial hemiplegic migraine genotypes, will further refine the early version of this overarching concept and reveal fully the intricacies of one of the most enduring mysteries that have puzzled humankind.

EPILOGUE

FOR THE MIGRAINE SUFFERER

He who rides a tiger cannot dismount – old Chinese proverb.

Why do I have this recurrent, nauseating and throbbing headache with aversion for light and sound? Am I weak in the head/brain? Or, is it my physical constitution? Why can't I drink alcohol without a headache? Why are my periods laced with headache? Why do I develop a headache during or after a workout, during laughing and talking, during coughing or straining at stools, or during shopping or partying? Is it gas in my abdomen (stomach for the lay person) that rises to my head to cause headache (a very frequent self-explanation offered by Asian/Indian patients)? Or, is it my hypertension? Or is it the low blood-pressure? Or is it just the stress of living? What about coffee and smoking cigarettes? Will systematic or rhythmic nasal breathing (called *Pranayama* in the ancient Indian system of medicine) help? Or, will acupuncture or other forms of alternative medicine help? Should I drink less or more water to stop these recurrent headaches? Does insomnia cause headache or the other way around? Why do I wake up with headaches? Are my headaches linked to my obesity or to my hypertension or to my genes? Should I undergo cardiac intervention or deep brain stimulation or botox therapy or other surgeries as a quick/permanent fix to my unending suffering? Or, am I going mad? Am I depressed because of headaches or do I develop headaches due to depression? Do I need psychiatric counseling? Will I have to live forever with this bolt-from-the-blue?

Should I participate in clinical trials and is there any assurance that I stand to benefit? Has science failed me or am I a spectacular one-of-a-kind failure? Shall I turn to grandma's cure for migraine? These and myriad other questions haunt every migraine sufferer worldwide.

Migraine sufferers asks such real-life questions to themselves as well as to their Physician / Neurologist / Ophthalmologist / Otorhinolaryngologist / Gynecologist / Psychiatrist in a desperate search for a logical and consistent answer. Migraine is both over-diagnosed and under-diagnosed. Since Physicians are usually the first point-of-contact, such questions are posed most often to the so-called non-specialists in Internal Medicine. Without an ounce of modesty and with quite a few grains of honesty, I state unhesitatingly that till a few years ago, I was never at ease with any explanation for migraine or its treatment that I gave to my patients. I believe that my colleagues handling their migraine patients are also still unable to give replies that are scientifically precise and subjectively satisfactory. We have been passing weak, disjointed conjectures and speculations as valid research-supported, particularly randomized-controlled-trial supported, explanations for occurrence of migraine to our patients. This book does not purport to be able to give a defensible explanation for this inquiry, but is an essential step in that direction. To be able to rationally satisfy the inquiries of our migraine patients, therapists must first convince themselves calmly and coldly, with a dispassionate hyper-critical focus on the constituents and the nature of migraine. Migraine therapists must no longer remain enthralled / enslaved by the 'wow' of either technology or RCTs. When technology is applied without foresight or when trials are conducted without insight or any care about their consequences, a sea of confusion ensues; currently, in medicine, no sea of confusion is larger or deeper than is migraine. No medical myth is more steeped in physiology, more believable, more logical, or more scientifically appealing than the myth of cortical spreading depression (CSD). For over fifty years, neurologists – scientists dominating migraine research – have believed in CSD as a Gospel truth. This generation of active headache researchers has ridden on the tiger of CSD and would not know what to believe in if CSD were to be finally disproved and abandoned. For such scientists getting off CSD means loss of a life-time's scientific conviction/integrity/public profile – much worse than being eaten-up alive by a tiger. We reap what we sow.

The transformation of migraine from a medical and literary curiosity and light-hearted upper-crust party-talk to a formal science is a fascinating saga by itself. As a medical point of discussion by the laity in the spoken or the printed word, migraine never lost its fascination or went out of vogue. Migraine is fiscally neutral and color-blind, striking equally the rich and the indigent, the celebrity and the riff-raff and the rabble, the white and the black and the brown races. All forms of alternative medicines, from acupuncture to homeopathy, profess to cure migraine with unparalleled sincerity. From a point where everyone knew everything that was knowable about migraine, we have come to the stage where the migraine expert knows nothing *definite* about migraine except the very obvious phenomenology. Migraine has two parts: easy (outer shell) and hard (inner core) – the inverse of a coconut. The easy part is the phenomenology that has been shaped into a giant, unwieldy classification system that, in turn, has been touted very frequently in major medical periodicals as the major advance of this generation. The hard part about migraine is its pathophysiology. Myths abound in the pathophysiology as well as the therapy of migraine, some created as late as in the twenty-first century. Wrapped up in serendipity and empiricism, migraine has defied the onslaught of technology and clinical trials to remain as impervious as it was since its first recognition over two thousand years ago. While theories and hypotheses abound, migraine has proved a classic medical mystery – one that Sherlock Holmes, the low-tech sleuth, would have been proud to unravel.

The study of adaptive mechanisms in migraine lays emphasis on what keeps migraine at bay, both in the migraine patient as well as in persons who never experience migraine in a lifetime. Like a veritable Trojan Horse -- beginning with vasopressin, the hormone that helps us to hold water -- operating at the heart of migraine pathophysiology, *adaptive mechanisms have crystallized a template upon which discrete and disparate laboratory observations can be brought to a focus that is both unifying as well as comprehensive.* Such a focus, if insightful and correct, should grow spontaneously – continuing to strengthen by addition of new facts and associations to the existing theoretical structure while meeting old and new challenges head-on. ***While it has given me a measure of intellectual pleasure in unfolding the concept of migraine adaptive mechanisms, nothing could delight me more than a sustained and devastating challenge to the concept by an individual or a school of experts.*** *The value of logic – and Karl Popper -- to science is incalculable. While no amount of evidence ever proves a case,* *any hypothesis might be disproved by a single piece of contradictory evidence – a shining beacon in the darkness of ignorance. **The mega-concept espoused herein is a paradoxical one, with no direct supporting data. I am, nevertheless, in constant search for evidences that might disprove my own theory of adaptive mechanisms in migraine. This is the other face of research; the quiet contemplation of things as they are, not as things ought to be in accordance with a preferred theory or conjecture or preconception. Such contemplation comes with the freedom to pursue truth without regard to cost or immediate utility or scientific standing. The privilege of theorizing (as also conducting clinical trials) carries with itself the onerous liability of dampening one's own enthusiasm and of acknowledging error. Watson and Crick (The Double helix)* teamed into a formidable research juggernaut on the basis of precisely such a philosophical approach.*** [498]

For the average migraine patient, the fierce debate among the experts about the origin (in the human body) of the disorder carries little meaning but is intimately related to the questions that the suffering generates. Even among the experts, it seems foolhardy to venture today that migraine might not arise from a perturbation (howsoever poorly understood) of the brain. Riding the tiger of *cortical spreading depression* – the most favored migraine theory – can only take us so far. For most humans, including medical scientists, philosophic commitment is a double-edged sword. *Even if, perchance, the error is recognized, the pre-commitment precludes public acceptance. Since long, nevertheless, the stalemate in understanding migraine is all too obvious.*

A new turn to the complex history of migraine was provided by the publication and dissemination of an abbreviated abstract of my concept of migraine in 1990 in the book, *Spirit of Enterprise, The 1990 Rolex Awards,* Buri International, Bern, Switzerland. I remain indebted to the essence of the Rolex Awards without which the present book could not have been conceived. A gigantic canvas was required to paint the true colors of migraine; such a canvas is not afforded by medical periodicals with the cynical-to-downright-hostile and anonymous peer-review system. *If I have climbed a personal Everest, it has been without oxygen, and more importantly, without gloves or footwear. Most critically, the uphill process included dogged refusal to buckle under severe peer-pressure tantamount to intellectual ridicule at almost every step.*[479][1,2] With due process of peer review in modern medical

---

[1] J.E. Riggs. Priority, rivalry, and peer review. J. Child Neurology. 1995;10:255-256.

journalism, my chances of getting to the first base of originality in migraine were no more than a distant dream or an elusive mirage. *I have a vintage collection of reviewers' vitriol, vitriol that strangely turbo-charged my crusade to set right the thinking of a very large group of primary headache researchers*. The evolution of my concept of migraine carries in its wake the funeral dirge for *cortical spreading depression* as a migraine mechanism. Some of my most valuable critiques as letters-to-the-Editor have still not been published even a decade after acceptance by the Editor. I had to virtually plead repeatedly to get my major reviews finally published much later after their acceptance. My detractors were experts in migraine clinging to their convictions (and that of their peers) at the expense of overpowering but contrary logic – a common human tendency. *Drummond Rennie put across this human frailty succinctly and superbly: peer review exists to keep egg off authors' faces*.[3]

I believe with total conviction that migraine neither originates in the brain nor is directly consequential to brain neuronal dysfunction. I framed my vision of migraine as arising from a perturbation of ocular hemodynamics in 2006 in Medical Hypotheses. The theory was met, not with any criticism or sarcasm, but with deafening silence – the surefire way, besides outright rejection, to castrate or obliterate originality. Once the sound and the fury and the swirling clouds of doubt have settled, migraine will be de-mystified and prove to be, in principle, scientifically as simple in nature as the microscope, the telephone, the motor-car, the airplane, the submarine or the space-module landing on Earth's moon and other planets of the solar system.

For any migraine (or cluster headache or chronic daily headache) patient contemplating participation in clinical trials, the chapter on PFO is an eye-opener and should be essential reading. As a scientist burdened with a different view of migraine, my most salient contribution to migraine research may well be restoration of the value of the patient as the end-point of scientific endeavors in this field.

In this madding and maddening quest, I had a possible advantage that I must disclose. My mother, my sister and her son, my wife, my son, and I myself all suffer from migraine. As a migraine-wounded therapist also

---

[2] D.F. Horrobin. Lancet 1996;348:1293-1295.
[3] S. Goldbeck-Wood. Br. Med. J. 1998;316:86.

surrounded by migraine patients in the family who jeered at me – and my pretensions of being a migraine researcher -- each time a migraine attack recurred amongst us, my thirst for the essence of migraine was unquenchable. I have learnt much about the philosophy and the science of both life and medicine from my migraine patients. Migraine is a protean, chameleon-like disorder that regularly dishes out lessons in humility to pretenders daring to unwrap its mystery or hoping to manage its victims. As if it had a life of its own, migraine reckons carefully the motive of both its seeker as well as the healer. In human endeavor, nothing can be more important than motive, a truism captured so eloquently by Denis P. Burkitt:

> Attitudes are more important than abilities.
> Motives are more important than methods.
> Character is more important than cleverness.
> Perseverance is more important than power.
> And the heart takes precedence over the head.[499]

Beyond knowledge lies wisdom, and beyond wisdom lurks faith. The slow dance between migraine-related knowledge, wisdom, and faith that began over two millennia ago appears to have quickened its pace. At the frontier of science, humans grapple with the occult and the unknown. Migraine is as occult as any disorder can be. Insight is a rare commodity in migraine, rarer than water in the desert. Genius is nothing but insight gifted from The Source. A select verse from Rumi, the mystic, sets the stage for this tango between the tangible and the intangible, this meandering between the measurable and the immeasurable:

> Since you have seen the dust, see the Wind.
> Since you have seen the foam, see the Ocean.
> Come, see it, for insight is the only thing in you that avails;
> the rest of you is a piece of fat and flesh.[500]

Across cultures, the urge to understand life itself as well as the ostensibly random bequeathement of originality or creative genius is a never-ending, never-fulfilled quest. ***Life and creative genius cannot be dissociated***.

> "What do you possess that was not given to you?
> If then you really received it as a gift,
> Why take the credit to yourself ?" -- Apostle Paul

"Life was there, a given thing;
The loan is reclaimed,
When the life is extinguished." -- Mirza Ghalib

"You would know in words that which you have always
known in thought.
You would touch with your fingers the naked body of your
dreams." -- Kahlil Gibran

"Can you, mating with heaven
Serve as the female part?
Can your learned head take leaven
From the wisdom of your heart?" – Lao Tzu (translated by Witter Bynner)

Carlo Rubbia (1934-), Director of CERN, affirms that scientific discovery is originally based on intuition, and is much closer to the creative process of the artist than readers of scientific papers realize.[4] *Where the primary intuition comes from, however, is pure mystery, and perhaps, fittingly so. The intellectual strength of science lies in its essentially subversive character.[5] The origin of inspired scientific intuition lies in the obscure subversive mental processes that refuse to accept compromises in knowledge that have passed as science for centuries or millennia. A Simple, Timeless Awareness[6] or the Timeless Original Mind[7] determines the final telluric instrument of unburdening, etching in temporal terms the push from the past and the pull from the future. In science and art, life's mega-illusion of being the doer is amplified manifold for the instrument. "It is not we who possess art; rather, it is art...that sometimes takes possession of people and in part manifests itself through them."— Andrei Donatovich Sinyavsky.*

---

[4] A. Storr. Lancet 1993; 341 (April 24):1062-1063.

[5] R. Horton. Lancet 1995; 346: 3.

[6] A. Huxley. The Perennial Philosophy. Triad Grafton Books: London, 1985.

[7] A. Watts. The Way of Zen, New York: Vintage, 1989.

With the publication of this volume, we now stand the cusp of a very exciting period in medical research insofar as the evolution of migraine as an entity is concerned. For scientists immersed in migraine research, the concept of adaptive mechanisms offers a huge conceptual leap. For migraine patients, a fuller comprehension of migraine dilutes the social stigma attached to the disorder as well as reduces exposure to therapeutic misadventures. If there is a 'weakness of constitution' in migraine, so is it in cancer and in coronary artery disease.

Vinod K. Gupta, M.D.
27 January, 2009

"I shall let the little that I have learnt go forth into the day in order that someone better than I may guess the truth, and in his work may prove and rebuke my error..." --- Albrecht Dürer.

REFERENCES

[1] Cutrer, F.M. (2006). Pathophysiology of migraine. *Semin. Neurol, 26*, 171-180.

[2] Goadsby, P.J., Lipton, R.B. and Ferrari, M.D. (2002). Migraine – current understanding and treatment. *N. Eng. J. Med, 346*, 257-270.

[3] Aurora, S. (2006). Botulinum toxin type A for the treatment of migraine. *Expert. Opin. Pharmacother, 7*, 1085-1095.

[4] Wilmshurst, P.T., Nightingale, S., Walsh, K.P., Morrison, W.L. (2005). Clopidogrel reduces migraine with aura after transcatheter closure of persistent foramen ovale and atrial septal defects. *Heart, 91*, 1173-1175.

[5] Afridi, S.K., Shields, K.G., Bhola, R. and Goadsby, P.J. (2006). Greater occipital nerve injection in primary headache syndromes – prolonged effects from a single injection. *Pain, 122*, 126-129.

[6] Jelinski, S.E., Becker, W.J., Christie, S.N., Giammarco, R., Mackie, G.F., Gawel, M.J., Eloff, A.G. and Magnusson J.E. (2006). Clinical features and pharmacological treatment of migraine patients referred to headache specialists in Canada. *Cephalalgia, 26*, 578-588.

[7] Edvinsson, L. and Uddman, R. (2005). Neurobiology in primary headaches. *Brain Res. Rev, 48*, 438-456.

[8] Pietrobon, D. (2005). Migraine: new molecular mechanisms. *Neuroscientist, 11*, 373-386. 9.

[9] Welch, K.M.A. (2005). Brain hyperexcitability: the basis for antiepileptic drugs in migraine prevention. *Headache, 45 (Suppl 1)*, S25-S32.

[10] Shields, K.G. and Goadsby, P.J. (2005). Propranolol modulates trigeminovascular responses in thalamic ventroposteromedial nucleus: a role in migraine? *Brain, 128*, 86-97.

[11] Goadsby, P.J. (2002). Neurovascular headache and a midbrain vascular malformation: evidence for a role of the brainstem in chronic migraine. *Cephalalgia, 22,* 107-111.

[12] Welch, M. (1998). The occipital cortex as a generator of migraine aura. *Cephalalgia, 18 (Suppl 22),* 15-21.

[13] Blau, J.N. (1992). Migraine: theories of pathogenesis. *Lancet, 339,* 1202-1207.

[14] Pearce, J.M.S. (1985). Is migraine explained by Leao's spreading depression? *Lancet, ii,* 763-766.

[15] Ayata, C., Jin, H., Kudo, C., Dalkara, T., Moskowitz, M.A. (2006). Suppression of cortical spreading depression in migraine prophylaxis. *Ann. Neurol, 59,* 652-661.

[16] Parsons, A.A. (2004). Cortical spreading depression: its role in migraine pathogenesis and possible therapeutic intervention strategies. *Curr. Pain Headache Rep, 8,* 410- 416.

[17] Welch, K.M.A. (1987). Migraine. A biobehavioral disorder. *Arch. Neurol, 44,* 323-327.

[18] Welch, K.M.A., D'Andrea, G., Tepley, N., Barkley, G. and Ramadan, N.M. (1990). The concept of migraine as a state of central neuronal hyperexcitability. *Neurol. Clin, 8,* 817-828.

[19] Gupta, V.K. (2006). Migrainous scintillating scotoma and headache is ocular in origin: a new hypothesis. *Med. Hypotheses, 66,* 454-460.

[20] Gupta, V. (2005). Migraine, cortical excitability, and evoked potentials: a clinico-pharmacological perspective. *Brain, 128,* E36.

[21] Gupta, V. (2006). Orbitofrontal cortex hypometabolism, medication overuse headache, substance abuse, and migraine: key pathophysiological issues. *Brain, 129,* E52. Full text/PDF available at: http://brain.oxfordjournals.org/cgi/reprint/129/7/E52?ijkey= 90InZaNWVxHtsZXandkeytype=ref

[22] Gupta, V.K. (2006). Migraine: "how" versus "what" of a disease process. *BMJ,* (8 February 2006). Available at: http://bmj.bmjjournals.com/cgi/eletters/332/7532/25#127734

[23] Edmeads, J. (1991). What is migraine? Controversy and stalemate in migraine pathophysiology. *J. Neurol, 238,* S2-S5.

[24] Headache Classification Subcommittee of the International Headache Society. (2004). The International Classification of Headache Disorders. 2nd edition. *Cephalalgia, 24(Suppl 1),* 9-160.

[25] Gupta, V.K. (2004). Magnesium therapy for migraine: do we need more trials or more reflection? *Headache, 44,* 445.

[26] Gupta, V.K. (2004). Randomized controlled trials: the hijacking of basic sciences by mathematical logic. *BMJ*, (6 July 2004). Available at: http://bmj.bmjjournals.com/ cgi/eletters/329/7456/2#65969

[27] Horton, R.C. and Kendall, M.J. (1991). Clinical pharmacology and therapeutics. *Postgrad Med J, 67*, 1042-1054.

[28] Feinstein, A.R. (1994). Clinical judgment revisited: the distractions of quantitative models. *Ann. Intern. Med, 120*, 799-805.

[29] Editorial. (1993). Does research make for better doctors? *Lancet, 342*, 1063-1064.

[30] Medawar, P.B. (1979). Advice to a young scientist. New York: Harper and Row.

[31] Peroutka, S.J. (2004). Migraine: a chronic sympathetic nervous system disorder. *Headache, 44*, 53-64.

[32] Charlton, B.G. (1992). Stress. *J. Med. Ethics, 18*, 156-159.

[33] Gupta, V.K. (2004). Sympathetic nervous system dysfunction in migraine: pearls and pitfalls in the theorizing process. *Headache, 44*, 841-842.

[34] Wall, P.D. and Melzack, R. (1989). *Textbook of Pain*, 2nd ed. New York: Churchill Livingstone.

[35] van Pragg, H.M., Lader, M.H., Rafaelsen, O.J. and Sachar, E.J. (1979). *Handbook of Biological Psychiatry*. New York: Marcel Dekker.

[36] Gupta, V.K. (2004). Stress, adaptation, and traumatic-event headaches: pathophysiologic and pharmacotherapeutic insights. *BMC Neurology*, (26 November 2004). Available at: *http://www.biomedcentral.com/1471-2377/4/17/comments#106454*

[37] Gupta, V.K. (1997). A clinical review of the adaptive potential of vasopressin in migraine. *Cephalalgia, 17*, 561-569.

[38] Willoughby, J.O. (1981). The pathophysiology of vegetative symptoms in migraine. *Lancet, ii*, 445-446.

[39] Poole, C.J.M. and Lightman, S.L. (1988). Inhibition of vasopressin secretion during migraine. *J. Neurol. Neurosurg. Psychiatry, 51*, 1441-1444.

[40] Drummond, P.D. and Granston, A. (2004). Facial pain increases nausea and headache during motion sickness in migraine sufferers. *Brain, 127*, 526-34.

[41] Cupini, L.M., Santorelli, F.M., Iani, C., Fariello, G. and Calabresi, P. (2003). Cyclic vomiting syndrome, migraine, and epilepsy: a common underlying disorder? *Headache, 43*, 407-409.

[42] Li, B.U. and Balint, J.P. (2000). Cyclic vomiting syndrome: evoluation in our understanding of a brain-gut disorder. *Adv. Pediatr, 47*, 117-160.

[43] Aurora, S.K., Kori, S.H., Barrodale, P., McDonald, S.A. and David Haseley, D. (2006). Gastric stasis in migraine: more than just a paroxysmal abnormality during a migraine attack. *Headache, 46,* 57-63.

[44] Hippocrates. (1859). In: Concerning Migraine. A. L. Allory. Thesis, Paris.

[45] Pearce, J.M. (1986). Historical aspects of migraine. *J. Neurol. Neurosurg. Psychiatry, 49,* 1097-1103.

[46] Campbell, J.K. (1990). Manifestations of migraine. *Neurol. Clin, 8,* 841-855.

[47] Blau, J.N. (1991). The clinical diagnosis of migraine: the beginning of therapy. *J. Neurol, 238(Suppl 1),* S6-S11.

[48] Rowe, J.W., Shelton, R.L., Helderman, J.H., Vetal, R.E. and Robertson, G.L. (1979). Influence of the emetic reflex on vasopressin release in man. *Kidney Int, 16,* 729-735.

[49] Valiquette, G. (1987). The neurohypophysis. *Neurol. Clin, 5,* 291-331.

[50] Faull, C.M., Rooke, P. and Bayliss, P.H. (1991). The effect of a highly specific serotonin agonist on osmoregulated vasopressin secretion in healthy man. *Clin. Endocrinol, 35,* 423-430.

[51] Gupta, V.K. (2004). Cyclic vomiting syndrome: anticipatory stress response in migraine? *Headache, 44,* 106.

[52] Gupta, V. (2005). Cyclical vomiting syndrome - migraine - vasopressin nexus: a new hypothesis for anticipatory nausea and vomiting. *BMC Pediatrics,* 5, 3. Available: *http://www.biomedcentral.com/1471-2431/5/3/comments/comments*

[53] Lance, J.W. and Anthony, M. (1971). Thermographic studies in vascular headache. *Med. J. Aust, 1,* 240-243.

[54] Hampton, K.K., Esack, A., Peatfield, R.C. and Grant, P.J. (1991). Elevation of plasma vasopressin in spontaneous migraine. *Cephalalgia, 11,* 249-250.

[55] Gupta, V.K. (1993). Does vasopressin serve a vasomotor adaptive function in migraine? *Cephalalgia, 13,* 220-221.

[56] Miranda-Cardenas, Y., Rojas-Piloni, G., Martínez-Lorenzana, G., Rodríguez-Jiménez, J., López-Hidalgo, M., Freund-Mercier, M.J. and Condés-Lara, M. (2006). Oxytocin and electrical stimulation of the paraventricular hypothalamic nucleus produce antinociceptive effects that are reversed by an oxytocin antagonist. *Pain, 122,* 182-189.

[57] Robinson, D.A., Wei, F., Wang, G.D., Li, P., Kim, S.J., Vogt, S.K., Muglia, L.J. and Zhuo, M. (2002). Oxytocin mediates stress-induced analgesia in adult mice. *J. Physiol. 540,* 593-606.

[58] Blau, J.N. (1982). Resolution of migraine attacks: sleep and the recovery phase. *J. Neurol. Neurosurg. Psychiatry, 45,* 223-6.

[59] Sahota, P.K. and Dexter, J.D. (1990). Sleep and headache syndromes: a clinical review. *Headache*, 30, 80-84.

[60] Kelman, L. and Rains, J.C. (2005). Headache and sleep: examination of sleep patterns and complaints in a large clinical sample of migraineurs. *Headache*, 45, 904-910.

[61] Peres, M.F.P., Stiles, M.A., Siow, H.C. and Silberstein, S,D. (2005). Excessive daytime sleepiness in migraine patients. *J. Neurol. Neurosurg. Psychiatry, 76,* 1467-1468.

[62] Gupta, V.K. (2005). Sleep remits and precipitates migraine: role of the monoaminergic-vasopressin system. *J. Neurol. Neurosurg. Psychiatry* (10 November 2005). Available at: http://jnnp.bmjjournals.com/cgi/eletters/76/10/1467.

[63] Dexter, J.D. (1979). The relationship between stage III + IV + REM sleep and arousals with migraine. *Headache, 19,* 364-369.

[64] Couch, J.R. and Hassanein, R.S. (1979). Amitriptyline in migraine prophylaxis. *Arch. Neurol, 36,* 695-699.

[65] Pearce, J.M.S. (1994). Headache. *J. Neurol. Neurosurg. Psychiatry, 57,* 134-143.

[66] Wilson, S. and Argyropoulos, S. (2005). Antidepressants and sleep. A qualitative review of the literature. *Drugs, 65,* 927-947.

[67] Kumar, K.K. (1988). Exercise for prophylaxis of migraine. *Headache, 28,* 228.

[68] van Gijn, J. (1987). Relief of common migraine by exercise. *J. Neurol. Neurosurg. Psychiatry, 50,* 1700-1701.

[69] Chen, T.C, Leviton, A., Edelstein, S. and Ellenberg, J.H. (1987). Migraine and other diseases in women of reproductive age. The influence of smoking on observed associations. *Arch. Neurol, 44,* 1024-1028.

[70] Stalnikowicz, R. (2006). Nicotine gum withdrawal and migraine headaches. *Eur. J. Emerg. Med, 13,* 247-248.

[71] Houezec, J.L. and Benowitz, N.L. (1991). Basic and clinical psychopharmacology of nicotine. *Clin. Chest. Med, 12,* 681-699.

[72] Simons, C.T., Cuellar, J.M., Moore, J.A., Pinkerton, K.E., Uyeminami, D., Carstens, M.I. and Carstens, E. (2005). Nicotinic receptor involvement in antinociception induced by exposure to cigarette smoke. *Neurosci. Lett, 389,* 71-76.

[73] Vincler, M. (2005). Neuronal nicotinic receptors as targets for novel analgesics. *Expert. Opin. Investig. Drugs, 14,* 1191-1198.

[74] Critchley, M. and Ferguson, F.R. (1933). Migraine. *Lancet, i,* 123-126.

[75]   Massey, E.W. (1977). Migraine during pregnancy. *Obstet Gynecol, 32,* 693-696.

[76]   Sances, G., Granella, F., Nappi, R.E., Fignon, A., Ghiotto, N., Polatti, F. and Nappi, G. (2003). Course of migraine during pregnancy and postpartum: a prospective study. *Cephalalgia, 23,* 197-205.

[77]   Barron, W.M. and Lindheimer, M,D. (1984). Renal sodium and water handling in pregnancy. *Obstet. Gynaecol. Annu, 13,* 35-69.

[78]   Okada, K., Ishikawa, S-E., Caramelo, C., Tsai, P. and Schrier, R.W. (1993). Enhancement of vascular action of arginine vasopressin by diminished xtracellular sodium concentration. *Kidney Int, 44,* 755-763.

[79]   Steiner, T.J., Scher, A.I., Stewart, W.F., Kolodner, K., Liberman, J. and Lipton, R.B. (2003). The prevalence and disability burden of adult migraine in England and their relationships to age, gender and ethnicity. *Cephalalgia, 23,* 519-527.

[80]   Yagi, K. (1992). Suppressive vasopressin response to emotional stress. *Jpn. J. Physiol, 42,* 681-703.

[81]   Onaka, T. and Yagi, K. (1988). Bimodal effects of noxious stimuli on vasopressin secretion in rats. *Neurosci. Res, 6,* 143-148.

[82]   Blau, J.N. and Thavapalan, M. (1988). Preventing migraine: a study of precipitating factors. *Headache, 28,* 481-483.

[83]   Lantéri-Minet, M., Radat, F., Chautard, M.H. and Lucas, C. (2005). Anxiety and depression associated with migraine: influence on migraine subjects' disability and quality of life, and acute migraine management. *Pain, 118,* 319-326.

[84]   Sanna, P.P., Folsom, D.P., Barizo, M.J., Hirsch, M.D., Melia, K.R., Maciejewski-Lenoir, D. and Bloom, F.E. (1993). Chronic ethanol intake decreases vasopressin mRNA content in the rat hypothalamus: a PCR study. *Brain Res. Mol. Brain Res, 19,* 241-245.

[85]   Anthony, M., Hinterberger, H. and Lance, J.W. (1967). Plasma serotonin in migraine and stress. *Arch. Neurol, 16,* 544-552.

[86]   Carroll, J.D. and Hilton, B.P. (1974). The effects of reserpine injection on methysergide treated control and migrainous subjects. *Headache, 14,* 149-156.

[87]   Alonso, G., Czernichow, P. and Assenmacher, I. (1985). Reserpine inhibits release of vasopressin from the neural lobe of the pituitary in dehydrated rats. *Cell Tiss. Res, 240,* 375-380.

[88]   Somerville, B.W. (1972). A study of migraine in pregnancy. *Neurology, 22,* 824-828.

[89] Callaghan, N. (1968). The migraine syndrome in pregnancy. *Neurology, 18,* 197-201.

[90] Lightman, S.L. (1993). Molecular insights into diabetes insipidus. *N. Engl. J. Med, 328,* 1562-1563.

[91] Kaiser, H.J. and Melenberg, O. (1993). Deterioration or onset of migraine under oestrogen replacement therapy in the menopause. *J. Neurol, 240,* 195-197.

[92] Genazzani, A.R., Petralgia, F., Volpe, A. and Facchinetti, F. (1985). Estrogen changes as a critical factor in modulation of central opioid tonus: possible correlations with postmenopausal migraine. *Cephalalgia, 5 (Supppl 2),* 211-214.

[93] Lance, J.W. (1992). Treatment of migraine. *Lancet,* 339, 1207-1209.

[94] Forsling, M.L. and and Aziz, L.A. (1983). Release of vasopressin in response to hypoxia and the effect of aminergic and opioid antagonists. *J. Endocrinol, 99, 77-86.*

[95] Lai, M., Loi, V., Pisano, M.R. and Del Zompo, M. (1997). Therapy of migraine by modulating dopamine hypersensitivity: its effect on mood and pain. *Int. J. Clin. Pharmacol. Res, 17,* 101-103.

[96] de Carolis, P., Tinuper, P. and Sacquegna, T. (1991). Migraine with aura and photosensitive epileptic seizures: a case report. *Cephalalgia, 11,* 151-153.

[97] Cerbo, R., Barbanti, P., Buzzi, M.G., Fabbrini, G., Brusa, L., Roberti, C., Zanette, E., and Lenzi, G.L. (1997). Dopamine hypersensitivity in migraine: role of the apomorphine test. *Clin. Neuropharmacol, 20,* 36-41.

[98] Nussey, S.S., Hawthorn, J., Page, S.R., Ang, V.T. and Jenkins, J.S. (1988). Responses of plasma oxytocin and arginine vasopressin to nausea induced by apomorphine and ipecacuanha. *Clin. Endocrinol, 28,* 297-304.

[99] Grant, P.J., Hughes, J.R., Dean, H.G., Davies, J.A. and Prentice, C.R. (1986). Vasopressin and catecholamine secretion during apomorphine-induced nausea mediate acute changes in haemostatic function in man. *Clin. Sci, 71,* 621-624.

[100] Colman, I., Brown, M.D., Innes, G.D., Grafstein, E., Roberts, T.E. and Rowe, B.H. (2004). Parenteral metoclopramide for acute migraine: meta-analysis of randomised controlled trials. *BMJ, 329,* 1369-73.

[101] Friedman, B.W., Corbo, J., Lipton, R.B., Bijur, P.E., Esses, D., Solorzano, C. and Gallagher, E.J. (2005). A trial of metoclopramide vs sumatriptan for the emergency department treatment of migraines. *Neurology, 64,* 463-468.

[102] Steardo, L., Iovino, M., Monteleone, P., Bevilacqua, M. and Norbiato, G. (1990). Evidence that cholinergic receptors of muscarinic type may

modulate vasopressin release induced by metoclopramide. *J. Neural. Transm. Gen. Sect, 82,* 213-217.

[103] Coiro, V., Capretti, L., Speroni, G., Volpi, R., Fagnoni, F., Bianconi, L., Schianchi, L., Caiazza, A. and Chinodera, P. (1989). Muscarinic cholinergic, but not serotoninergic mediation of arginine vasopressin response to metoclopramide in man. *Clin. Endocrinol, 31,* 491-498.

[104] Peroutka, S.J. (1997). Dopamine and migraine. *Neurology, 49,* 650-656.

[105] Duke-Elder, S. (1968). The physiology of the eye and of vision. System of Ophthalmology, vol. 4. London: Henry Kimpton.

[106] Gondim, E.L., Liu, J.H., Costa, V.P. and Weinreb, R.N. (2001). Exogenous vasopressin influences intraocular pressure via the V(1) receptors. *Curr. Eye Res, 22,* 295-303.

[107] Gupta, V.K. (2005). Intraocular pressure, systemic blood pressure, and headache: occult pathophysiological link? *Br J Ophthalmol* (21 December 2005). Available at: http://bjo.bmjjournals.com/cgi/eletters/89/3/284

[108] Lips, C.J., Lentjes, E.G. and Höppener, J.W. (2003). The spectrum of carcinoid tumours and syndromes. *Ann. Clin. Biochem, 40,* 612-627.

[109] Mathew, N.T., Tietjen, G.E. and Lucker, C. (1996). Serotonin syndrome complicating migraine pharmacotherapy. *Cephalalgia, 16,* 323-327.

[110] Kuritsky, A., Ziegler, D.K. and Hassanein, R. (1981). Vertigo, motion sickness and migraine. *Headache, 21,* 227-231.

[111] Neuhauser, H. and Lempert T. (2004). Vertigo and dizziness related to migraine: a diagnostic challenge. *Cephalalgia,* 24, 83-81.

[112] von Brevern, M., Zeise, D., Neuhauser, H., Clarke, A.H. and Lempert, T. (2005). Acute migrainous vertigo: clinical and oculographic findings. *Brain, 128,* 365-374.

[113] Gupta, V.K. (2005). Motion sickness is linked to nystagmus-related trigeminal brain stem input: a new hypothesis. *Med. Hypotheses, 64,* 1177-1181.

[114] Marchioro, G., Azzarello, G., Viviani, F., Barbato, F., Pavanetto, M., Rosetti, F., Pappagallo, G.L. and Vinante, O. (2000). Hypnosis in the treatment of anticipatory nausea and vomiting in patients receiving cancer chemotherapy. *Oncology, 59,* 100-104.

[115] Franceschini, R., Leandri, M., Cataldi, A., Bruno, E., Corsini, G., Rolandi, E. and Barreca, T. (1995). Raised plasma arginine vasopressin concentrations during cluster headache attacks. *J. Neurol. Neurosurg. Psychiatry, 59,* 381-383.

[116] Gupta, V.K. (2006). Cluster headache: Key pathophysiological issues. *J Neurol Neurosurg Psychiatry* (2 March 2006). Available at: http://jnnp.bmjjournals.com/cgi/ eletters/jnnp.2005.081158v1#869

[117] Blau, J.N. (1993). Behaviour during a cluster headache. *Lancet, 342,* 723-725.

[118] Markley, H.G. and Buse, D.C. (2006). Cluster headache: myths and the evidence. *Curr. Pain Headache Rep, 10,* 137-141.

[119] Peatfield, R. (1988). Drugs and the treatment of migraine. *Trends Pharmacol. Sci, 9,* 141-145.

[120] Lobzin, V.S. and Vasil'ev, N.S. (1989). Lechenie migreni vazopressinom. *Zh. Nevropatol. Psikhiatr, 1,* 54-58.

[121] Gupta, V.K. (2005). Recurrent syncope, hypotension, asthma, and migraine with aura: role of metoclopramide. *Headache, 45,* 1413-1415.

[122] Buschmann, J., Leppla-Wollsiffer, G., Nemeth, N., Nelson, K., and Kirsten, R. (1996). Migraine patients show increased platelet vasopressin receptors. *Headache, 36,* 586–588.

[123] Agarwal, K.C. (1993). Modulation of vasopressin actions on human platelets by plasma adenosine and theophylline: gender differences. *J. Cardiovasc. Pharmacol, 21,* 1012–1018.

[124] Peatfield, R.C., Hampton, K.K. and Grant, P.J. (1988). Plasma vasopressin levels in induced migraine attacks. *Cephalalgia, 8,* 55-57.

[125] Kim, M.S., Chey, W.D., Owyang, C. and Hasler, W.L. (1997). Role of plasma vasopressin as a mediator of nausea and gastric slow wave dysrhythmias in motion sickness. *Am. J. Physiol. Gastrointest. Liver Physiol, 272,* G853-G862.

[126] Chen, J.D., Qian, L., Ouyang, H. and Yin, J. (2003). Gastric electrical stimulation with short pulses reduces vomiting but not dysrhythmias in dogs. *Gastroenterology. 124,* 401-409.

[127] Ikegaya, Y. and Matsuki, N. (2002). Vasopressin induces emesis in *Suncus murinus. Jpn. J. Pharmacol, 89,* 324-326.

[128] Gupta, V.K. (2004). Conceptual divide between adaptive and pathogenetic phenomena in migraine: nausea and vomiting. *Brain, 127,* E18.

[129] Durlach, J., Pagès, N., Bac, P., Bara, M. and Guiet-Bara, A. (2005). Headache due to photosensitive magnesium depletion. *Magnes. Res, 18,* 109-122.

[130] Trauninger, A., Pfund, Z., Koszegi, T. and Czopf, J. (2002). Oral magnesium load test in patients with migraine. *Headache, 42,* 114-119.

[131] Gallai, V., Sarchielli, P., Mozucci, P. and Abritti, G. (1993). Red blood cell magnesium levels in migraine patients. *Cephalalgia, 13,* 74-81.

[132] Mauskop, A., Altura, B.T., Cracco, R.Q. and Altura, B.M. (1993). Deficiency in serum ionized magnesium but not total magnesium in patients with migraines. *Headache, 33,* 135-138.

[133] Thomas, J., Thomas, E. and Tomb, E. (1992). Serum and erythrocyte magnesium concentrations and migraine. *Magnes Res, 5,* 127-130.

[134] Schoenen, J., Sianard-Gainko, J. and Lenaerts, M. (1991). Blood magnesium levels in migraine. *Cephalalgia, 11,* 97-99.

[135] Boska, M.D., Welch, K.M., Barker, P.B., Nelson, J.A. and Schultz, L. (2002). Contrast in cortical magnesium, phospholipids and energy metabolism between migraine syndromes. *Headache, 42,* 114-119.

[136] Lodi, R., Iotti, S., Cortelli, P., Pierangeli, G., Cevoli, S., Clementi, V., Soriani, S., Montagna, P. and Barbiroli, B. (2001). Deficient energy metabolism is associated with low free magnesium in the brains of patients with migraine and cluster headache. *Brain Res. Bull, 54,* 437-431.

[137] Ramadan, N.M., Halvorson, H., Vandelinde, A., Levine, S., Helpern, J.A. and Welch, K.M.A. (1989). Low brain magnesium in migraine. *Headache, 29,* 590-593.

[138] Frank, L.R., Olson, C.M., Shuler, K.B. and Gharib, S.F. (2004). Intravenous magnesium for acute benign headache in the emergency department: a randomized double-blind placebo-controlled trial. *Can. J. Emerg. Med, 6,* 327-32

[139] Wang, F., Van Den Eeden, S.K., Ackerson, L.M., Salk, S.E., Reince, R.H. and Elin, R.J. (2003). Oral magnesium oxide prophylaxis of frequent migrainous headache in children: a randomized, double-blind, placebo-controlled trial. *Headache, 43,* 601- 610.

[140] Corbo, J., Esses, D., Bijur, P.E., Iannaccone, R. and Gallagher, E.J. (2001). Randomized clinical trial of intravenous magnesium sulfate as an adjunctive medication for emergency department treatment of migraine headache. *Ann. Emerg. Med, 38,* 621-627.

[141] Pfaffenrath, V., Weseley, P., Meyer, C., Isler, H.R., Evers, S., Grotemeyer, K.H., Taneri, Z., Soyka, D., G"bel, H. and Fischer, M. (1996). Magnesium in the prophylaxis of migraine: a double blind placebo-controlled trial. *Cephalalgia, 16,* 346-340.

[142] Mauskop, A., Altura, B.T., Cracco, R.Q. and Altura, B.M. (1996). Intravenous magnesium sulfate rapidly alleviates headaches of various types. *Headache, 36,* 154-160.

[143] Gupta, V.K. (2004). Magnesium therapy for migraine: do we need more trials or more reflection? *Headache, 44,* 445-446.

[144] Gupta, V.K. (2004). Non-lateralizing brain PET changes in migraine: phenomenology versus pharmacology? *Brain, 127,* E12.

[145] Mishima, K., Takeshima, T., Shimomura, T., Okada, H., Kitano, A., Takahashi, K. and Nakashima, K. (1997). Platelet ionized magnesium, cyclic AMP, and cyclic GMP levels in migraine and tension-type headache. *Headache, 37,* 561-564.

[146] Johnson, S. (2001). The multifaceted and widespread pathology of magnesium deficiency. *Med. Hypotheses, 56,* 163-170.

[147] Wong, E.T., Rude, R.K., Singer, F.R. and Shaw, S.T. (1983). A high prevalence of hypomagnesemia and hypermagnesemia in hospitalized patients. *Am. J. Clin. Pathol, 79,* 348-352.

[148] Thomsen, L.L., Kruuse, C., Iversen, H.K. and Olesen, J. (1994). A nitric oxide donor (nitroglycerine) triggers genuine migraine attacks. *Eur. J. Neurol., 1,* 73-80.

[149] Gupta, V.K. (1996). Does magnesium supplementation have any role in acute myocardial infarction? No. *Cardiovasc. Drugs Ther., 10,* 303-305.

[150] Antman, E.M., Seelig, M.S., Fleischmann, K., Lau, J., Kuntz, K., Berkey, C.S. and McIntosh, M.W. (1996). Magnesium in acute myocardial infarction: scientific, statistical, and economic rationale for its use. *Cardiovasc. Drugs Ther., 10,* 297-301.

[151] Yusuf, S. and Flather, M. Editorial. Magnesium in acute myocardial infarction. ISIS 4 provides no grounds for its use. *Br. Med. J., 310,* 751-752.

[152] Egger, M. and Smith, G.D. (1995). Misleading meta-analysis. Lessons from an "effective, safe, simple" intervention that wasn't. *Br. Med. J.,* 310, 752-754.

[153] Magnesium in Coronaries (MAGIC) Trial Investigators. (2002). Early administration of intravenous magnesium to high-risk patients with acute myocardial infarction in the Magnesium in Coronaries (MAGIC) Trial: a randomised controlled trial. *Lancet, 360,* 1189-96.

[154] Antman, E.M. (2002). Magnesium in coronaries. The MAGIC study. Program and abstracts of the European Society of Cardiology Congress, August 31-September 4, 2002; Berlin, Germany.

[155] Ko, S.H., Lim, H.R., Kim, D.C., Han, Y.J., Choe, H. and Song, H.S. (2001). Magnesium sulfate does not reduce postoperative analgesic requirements. *Anesthesiology, 95,* 640-646.

[156] Gupta, V.K. (2004). Re: Re: Randomized controlled trials: the mythical hypomagnesaemia - intrinsic noradrenergic activation - cortical spreading depression nexus in migraine. *BMJ.* Online (8 July 2004). Available at: http://bmj. bmjjournals.com/ cgi/eletters/329/7456/2#65969

[157] Roberts, J.M., Villar, J. and Arulkumaran, S. (2002). Preventing and treating eclamptic seizures. Magnesium sulphate is effective and recommended for use. *BMJ, 325*, 609-610.

[158] Duley, L. (2005). Evidence and practice: the magnesium sulphate story. *Best Pract. Res. Clin. Obstet. Gynae, 19*, 57-74.

[159] Sadeh, M. (1989). Action of magnesium sulphate in the treatment of preeclampsia-eclampsia. *Stroke, 20*, 1273-1275.

[160] Esen, F., Erdem, T., Aktan, D., Orhan, M., Kaya, M., Eraksoy, H., Cakar, N. and Telci, L. (2005). Effect of magnesium sulfate administration on blood-brain barrier in a rat model of intraperitoneal sepsis: a randomized controlled experimental study. *Crit. Care, 9*, R18-23.

[161] Kaya M, Gulturk S, Elmas I, Kalayci, R., Arican, N., Kocyildiz, Z.C., Kucuk, M., Yorulmaz, H. and Sivas, A. (2004). The effects of magnesium sulfate on blood- brain barrier disruption caused by intracarotid injection of hyperosmolar mannitol in rats. *Life Sci, 76*, 201-212.

[162] Esen, F., Erdem, T., Aktan, D., Kalayci, R., Cakar, N., Kaya, M. and Telci, L. (2003). Effects of magnesium administration on brain edema and blood-brain barrier breakdown after experimental traumatic brain injury in rats. *J. Neurosurg. Anesthesiol, 15*, 119-125.

[163] Kaya, M., Küçük, M., Kalayci, R.B., Cimen, V., Gürses, C., Elmas, I. and Arican, N. (2001). Magnesium sulfate attenuates increased blood-brain barrier permeability during insulin-induced hypoglycemia in rats. *Can. J. Physiol. Pharmacol, 79*, 793-798.

[164] Altura, B.T. and Altura, B.M. (1982). The role of magnesium in etiology of strokes and cerebrovasospasm. *Magnesium, 1*, 277-291.

[165] Seelig, M. (1989). Cardiovascular consequences of magnesium deficiency and loss: pathogenesis, prevalence and manifestations—magnesium and chloride loss in refractory potassium repletion. *Am. J. Cardiol, 63*, 4G-21G.

[166] Blau, J.N. (1992). The challenge of unexplained diseases: migraine. *J. Roy. Soc. Med, 85*, 593-594.

[167] Blau, J.N. (1991) Migraine postdromes: symptoms after attacks. *Cephalalgia, 11*, 229-231.

[168] Jarcho S. (1967). General Grant's headache. Bull. N Y Acad. Sc.i 43, 1224-1226.

[169] O'Brien, S. (1991). *Ulysses S. Grant. iPictureBooks, Inc.* Date published: 01/14/2003. Excerpt available at: http://www.ereader.com/product/book/excerpt/10005?book= Ulysses_S._Grant

[170] Friedman, A.P. (1985). Headache. In: Baker, A.B. and Joynt, R.J. (eds) *Clinical Neurology,* rev. ed. Philadelphia: Harper and Row, 13:1-50.

[171] Gupta, V. (2006). Silent or non-clinical infarct-like lesions in the posterior circulation territory in migraine: brain hypoperfusion or hyperperfusion? *Brain, 129,* E39. Full Text: PDF: *http://brain.oxfordjournals.org/cgi/ reprint/129/1/ E39?ijkey= KCcr3z28Z mDWzywandkeytype=ref*

[172] Poole, C.J.M. Migraine. (1986). *Br. J. Hosp. Med, 36,* 90-93.

[173] Satel, S.L. and Gawin, F.H. (1989). Migrainelike headache and cocaine use. *JAMA, 261,* 2995-2996.

[174] Dhuna, A., Pascaul-Leone, A. and Belgrade, M. (1991). Cocaine-related vascular headaches. *J. Neurol. Neurosurg. Psychiatry, 54,* 803-806.

[175] Couturier, E.G.M., Hering, R. and Steiner, T.J. (1992). Weekend attacks in migraine patients: caused by caffeine withdrawal? *Cephalalgia, 12,* 99-100.

[176] Brewerton, T.D., Murphy, D.L., Mueller, E.A. and Jimerson, D.C. (1988). Induction of migraine-like headaches by the serotonin agonist m-chlorophenylpiperazine. *Clin. Pharmacol. Ther, 43,* 605-609.

[177] Shulman, B.H. Psychiatric aspects of headache. (1991). *Med. Clin. North Am, 75,* 707-715.

[178] Haas, D.C. (2004). Traumatic-event headaches. *BMC Neurology, 4,* 17.

[179] Rabkin, R., Stables, D.P., Levin, N.W. and Suzman, M.M. (1966). The prophylactic value of propranolol in angina pectoris. *Am. J. Cardiol, 18,* 370-383.

[180] Gupta, V.K. (2006). Botulinum toxin: a treatment for migraine? A systematic review. *Pain Med, 7,* 386-394.

[181] Gupta, V.K. (2006). Interatrial shunt associated migraine: serendipity, empiricism, hope, or hype? *Stroke, 37,* 2212.

[182] Stratakis, C.A. and Chrousos, G.P. (1995). Neuroendocrinology and pathophysiology of the stress system. *Ann. N Y Acad. Sci, 771,* 1-18.

[183] Shechter, A., Stewart, W.F., Silberstein, S.D. and Lipton, R.B. (2002). Migraine and autonomic nervous system function: a population-based, case-control study. *Neurology, 58,* 422-427.

[184] Mathias, C.J., and Bannister, R.B. (1999). Investigation of autonomic disorders. In: C. J. Mathias, and R.B. Bannister (Eds.) *Autonomic Failure: A Textbook of Clinical Disorders of the Autonomic nervous System* (4th ed. 169-195). New York: Oxford University Press.

[185] Mascia, A., Áfra, J. and Schoenen, J. (1998). Dopamine and migraine: a review of pharmacological, biochemical, neurophysiological, and therapeutic data. *Cephalalgia* 18 (4), 174-182.

[186] Hsu, L.K.G., Crisp, A.H., Kalucy, R.S., Koval, J., Chen, C.N., Carruthers, M. and Zilkha, K.J. (1977). Early morning migraine. Nocturnal plasma

levels of catecholamines, tryptophan, glucose and free-fatty acids and sleep encephalographs. *Lancet, ii,* 447-451.

[187] Kopera, H. (1978). Anticholinergic and blood pressure effects of mianserin, amitriptyline and placebo. *Br. J. Clin. Pharmacol, 5 (Suppl 1),* 29S-34S.

[188] Croos, R., Thirumalai, S., Hassan, S., Da, J. and Davis, R. (2005). Citalopram associated with acute angle-closure glaucoma: case report. *BMC Ophthalmology, 5,* 23.

[189] Second round-table medical therapy of glaucoma. (1975). *Doc. Ophthalmol,* 33, 245-269.

[190] McCall, R.B. and Humphrey, S.J. (1982). Involvement of serotonin in the central regulation of blood pressure: evidence for a facilitating effect on sympathetic nerve activity. *J. Pharm. Exp. Ther, 222,* 96-102.

[191] Antonaccio, M.J. and Taylor, D.G. (1977). Reduction in blood pressure, sympathetic nerve discharge and centrally evoked pressor responses by methysergide in anesthetized cats. *Eur. J. Pharmacol, 21,* 331-338.

[192] Krootila, K., Oksala, O., Zschauer, A., Palkama, A. and Uusitalo, H. (1992). Inhibitory effect of methysergide on calcitonin gene-related peptide-induced vasodilatation and ocular irritative changes in the rabbit. *Br. J. Pharmacol, 106,* 404- 408.

[193] Abelson, M.B., Gilbert, C.M. and Smith, L.M. (1988). Sustained reduction of intraocular pressure in humans with the calcium channel blocker verapamil. *Am. J. Ophthalmol., 105,* 155-159.

[194] Yu, W. and Horowitz, SH. (2003). Treatment of sporadic hemiplegic migraine with calcium-channel blocker verapamil. *Neurology, 60,* 120-121.

[195] Silberstein, S.D. and Young, W.B. (1995). Migraine aura and prodrome. *Semin. Neurol., 15,* 175-182.

[196] Solomon, G.D. (1989). Verapamil in migraine prophylaxis--a five-year review. *Headache, 29,* 425-427.

[197] McArthur, J.C., Marek, K., Pestronk, A., McArthur, J. and Peroutka, S.J. (1989). Nifedipine in the prophylaxis of classic migraine: a crossover, double-masked, placebo-controlled study of headache frequency and side effects. *Neurology, 1989,* 284-286.

[198] Kelly, S.P. and Walley, T.J. (1988). Effect of the calcium antagonist nifedipine on intraocular pressure in normal subjects. *Br. J. Ophthalmol., 72,* 216-218.

[199] Mekki, Q.A., Hassan, S.M. and Turner, P. (1983). Bromocriptine lowers IOP without affecting blood pressure. *Lancet, i,* 1250.

[200] Gupta, V.K. (2006). Systemic hypertension, headache, and ocular hemodynamics: a new hypothesis. *MedGenMed, 8(3)*, (Posted 09/12/06). Available at: http://www.medscape.com/ viewarticle/542682_1.

[201] Yankovsky, A.E. and Kuritsky, A. (2003). Transformation into daily migraine with aura following transcutaneous atrial septal defect closure. *Headache, 43*, 496-498.

[202] Mortelmans, K., Post, M., Thijs, V., Herroelen, L., and Budts, W. (2005). The influence of percutaneous atrial septal defect closure on the occurrence of migraine. *Eur. Heart J, 26*, 1533-1537.

[203] Azarbal, B., Tobis, J., Suh, W., Chan, V., Dao, C. and Gaster, R. (2005). Association of interatrial shunts and migraine headaches. Impact of transcatheter closure. *J. Am. Coll. Cardiol, 45*, 489-492.

[204] Gupta, V.K. (2006). Closure of ASD: what aggravates the migrainous diathesis? *Eur. Heart J., 27*, 1756-1757.

[205] Gupta, V.K. (2005). PFO / ASD closure and migraine: searching the rationale for the procedure. *J. Am. Coll. Cardiol., 46*, 737-738.

[206] Tsimikas, S. (2005). Transcatheter closure of patent foramen ovale for migraine prophylaxis. Hope or hype? *J. Am. Coll. Cardiol, 45*, 496-498. [Free Full Text]

[207] Gupta V.K. (2005). Clopidogrel and atrial shunt closure for migraine: why is migraine aggravated immediately? *Heart* (13 December 2005). Available at: http://heart.bmjjournals.com/cgi/eletters/91/9/1173#869.

[208] Gupta, V.K. (2004). Closure of atrial septal defect and migraine. *Headache, 44*, 291- 292.

[209] Weerasuriya, K., Patel, L. and Turner, P. (1982). β-adrenoceptor blockade and migraine. *Cephalalgia, 2*, 33-45.

[210] Nanda, R.N., Johnson, R.H., Gray, J., Keogh, H.J. and Melville, I.D. (1978). A double-blind trial of acebutolol for migraine prophylaxis. *Headache, 18*, 20-22.

[211] Ekbom, K. and Zetterman, M. (1977). Oxprenolol in the treatment of migraine. *Acta. Neurol. Scand., 56*, 181-184.

[212] Ekbom, K. (1975). Alprenolol for migraine prophylaxis. *Headache, 15*, 129-132.

[213] Juang, K.D., Wang, S.J., Fuh, J.L., Lu, S.R. and Su, T.P. (2000). Comorbidity of depressive and anxiety disorders in chronic daily headache and its subtypes. *Headache, 40*, 818-823.

[214] Ossipova, V.V., Kolosova, O.A. and Vein, A.M. (1999). Migraine associated with panic attacks. *Cephalalgia, 19*, 728-731.

[215] Marazzti, D., Toni, C., Pedri, S., Bonuccelli, U., Pavese, N., Lucetti, C., Nuti, A., Muratorio, A. and Cassano, G.B. (1999). Prevalence of headache syndromes in panic disorder. *Int. Clin. Psychopharmacol, 14,* 247-251.

[216] Ying, M., Hui-chun, Li., Lei-lei Z. and Hua-liang, Y. (2006). Hemodynamic changes in depressive patients. *J. Zhejiang. Univ. Sci. B, 7,* 133-137.

[217] Alm, A. and Wickstrom, C.P. (1980). Effects of systemic and topical administration of metoprolol on intraocular pressure in healthy subjects. *Acta. Ophthalmol., 58,* 740-747.

[218] Krieglstein, G.K. (1978). The effect of metoprolol on IOP (Abstract). *Klin. Monatsbl. Augenheilkd, 173,* 632-7.

[219] Bonomi, L., Perfetti, S., Noya, E., Bellucci, R. and Massa, F. (1979). Comparison of the effects of nine beta-adrenergic blocking agents on intraocular pressure in rabbits. *Graefe's Archive for Clinical and Experimental Ophthalmology, 210,* 1-8.

[220] Bonomi, I. and Steindler, P. (1975). Effect of pindolol on intraocular pressure. *Br. J. Ophthalmol, 59,* 301-303.

[221] Siegner, S.W., Netland, P.A., Schroeder, A. and Ericksen, K.A. (2000). Effect of calcium channel blockers alone and in combination with antiglaucoma medications on intraocular pressure in the primate eye. *J. Glaucoma, 9,* 334-339.

[222] Estermann, S., Daepp, G-C., Cattapan-Ludewig, K., Berkhoff, M., Frueh, B.E. and Goldblum, D. (2006). Effect of oral donepezil on intraocular pressure in normotensive Alzheimer patients. *J. Ocul. Pharm. Ther, 22,* 62-67.

[223] Aygun, D., Altintop, L., Doganay, Z., Guven, H. and Baydin, A. (2003). Electrocardiographic changes during migraine attacks. *Headache, 43,* 861-866.

[224] Gupta, V.K. (2004). Parasympathetic hyperfunction during migraine attacks. *Headache, 44,* 730-731.

[225] Gupta, V.K. (2006). Role of parasympathetic nervous system and migraine: changing perspective. *Headache.* (In press).

[226] Yarnitsky, D., Goor-Aryeh, I., Bajwa, Z.H., Ransil, B.I., Cutrer, F.M., Sottile, A. and Burstein, R. (2003). 2003 Wolff Award: Possible parasympathetic contributions to peripheral and central sensitization during migraine. *Headache, 43,* 704-714.

[227] Avnon, Y., Nitzan, M., Sprecher, E., Rogowski, Z. and Yarnitsky, D. (2004). Autonomic asymmetry in migraine: augmented parasympathetic activation in left unilateral migraineurs. *Brain, 127,* 2099-2108.

[228] Peroutka, S.J. (2004). Re: A sympathetic view of "2003 Wolff Award: Possible parasympathetic contributions to peripheral and central sensitization during migraine". *Headache, 44,* 731-732.

[229] Besson, M., Brook, P., Chizh, B.A. and Pickering, A.E. (2005). Tactile allodynia in patients with postherpetic neuralgia: lack of change in skin blood flow upon dynamic stimulation. *Pain, 117,* 154-161.

[230] Samuelsson, M., Leffler, A.S. and Hansson, P. (2005). Dynamic mechanical allodynia: on the relationship between temporo-spatial stimulus parameters and evoked pain in patients with peripheral neuropathy. *Pain, 115,* 264-272.

[231] Greenspan, J.D., Ohara, S., Sarlani, E. and Lenz, F.A. (2004). Allodynia in patients with post-stroke central pain (CPSP) studied by statistical quantitative sensory testing within individuals. *Pain, 109,* 357-366.

[232] Jørum, E., Warncke, T. and Stubhaug, A. (2003). Cold allodynia and hyperalgesia in neuropathic pain: the effect of N-methyl-D-aspartate (NMDA) receptor antagonist ketamine--a double- blind, cross-over comparison with alfentanil and placebo. *Pain, 101,* 229-235.

[233] Witting, N., Kupers, R.C., Svensson, P., Arendt-Nielsen, L., Gjedde, A. and Jensen, T.S. (2001). Experimental brush-evoked allodynia activates posterior parietal cortex. *Neurology*, 57, 1817-24.

[234] Burstein, R., Collins, B. and Jakubowski, M. (2004). Defeating migraine pain with triptans: a race against the development of cutaneous allodynia. *Ann. Neurol*, 55, 19-26.

[235] Gupta, V.K. (2006). Pre-emptive / early intervention with triptans in migraine: hope, hype, and hazard. *Int. J. Clin. Pract.* (in press).

[236] Simons, C.T., Cuellar, J.M., Moore, J.A., Pinkerton, K.E., Uyeminami, D., Carstens, M.I. and Carstens, E. (2005). Nicotinic receptor involvement in antinociception induced by exposure to cigarette smoke. *Neurosci. Lett, 389,* 71-6.

[237] Vincler M. (2005). Neuronal nicotinic receptors as targets for novel analgesics. *Expert Opin. Investig. Drugs, 14,* 1191-1198.

[238] Nicolodi, M., Galeotti, N., Ghelardini, C., Bartolini, A. and Sicuteri, F. (2002). Central cholinergic challenging of migraine by testing second-generation anticholinesterase drugs. *Headache, 42,* 596-602.

[239] Yamamura, H., Malick, A., Chamberlin, N.L. and Burstein, R. (1999). Cardiovascular and neuronal responses to head stimulation reflect central sensitization and cutaneous allodynia in a rat model of migraine. *J. Neurophysiol, 81,* 479-93.

[240] Cruickshank, J,M. (1980). The clinical importance of cardio-selectivity and lipophilicity in betablockers. *Am. Heart J, 100,* 160-178.

[241] Stensrud, P. and Sjaastad, O. (1980). Comparative trial of tenormin (atenolol) and inderal (propranolol) in migraine. *Headache, 20,* 204-207.

[242] Johannsson V, Nilsson LR, Widelius T, Jäverfalk T, Hellman P, Åkesson J-Å, Olerud, B., Gustafsson, C-L., Raak, A., Sandhal, G., Tilling, B., Almkvist, G. and Troein, M. (1987). Atenolol in migraine prophylaxis: a double-blind cross-over multicentre study. *Headache,* 27, 372-374.

[243] Forssman, B., Lindblad, C.J. and Zbomikova, V. (1983). Atenolol for migraine prophylaxis. *Headache, 23,* 188-190.

[244] Kowacs, P.A. and Werneck, L.C. (1996). Atenolol prophylaxis in migraine secondary to an arteriovenous malformation. *Headache, 36,* 625-627.

[245] Emilien, G. and Maloteaux, J.M. (1998). Current therapeutic uses and potential of beta-adrenoceptor agonists and antagonists. *Eur. J. Clin. Pharmacol, 53,* 389-404.

[246] Andersson, K.E. and Vinge, E. (1990). Beta-adrenoceptor blockers and calcium antagonists in the prophylaxis and treatment of migraine. *Drugs,* 39, 355-373.

[247] Sudilovsky, A, Elkind, A.H., Ryan, R.E. Sr, Saper, J.R., Stern, M.A. and Meyer, J.H. (1987). Comparative efficacy of nadolol and propranolol in the management of migraine. *Headache, 27,* 421-426.

[248] Olerud, B., Gustavsson, C.L. and Furberg, B. (1986). Nadolol and propranolol in migraine management. *Headache, 26,* 490-493.

[249] Agnoli, A. (1988). The classification of calcium antagonists by the WHO expert committee: relevance in neurology. *Cephalalgia, 8 (Suppl 8),* 7-10.

[250] Gupta, V.K. (2006). Topiramate for migraine prophylaxis: addressing the blood-brain barrier related pharmacokinetic-pathophysiological disconnect. *Int. J. Clin. Pract, 60,* 367-368.

[251] Gupta, V.K. (2006). Pharmacotherapeutics of migraine and the blood-brain barrier serendipity, empiricism, hope, and hype. *MedGenMed, 8,* 89. Available at: http://medgenmed.medscape.com/viewarticle/536453 (Accessed September 29, 2006).

[252] Popper, K.P. (1959). The Logic of Scientific Discovery. (English Translation). London: Hutchinson.

[253] Haas, D.C. and Sheehe, P.R. (2004). Dextroamphetamine pilot crossover trials and n of 1 trials in patients with chronic tension-type and migraine headache. *Headache, 44,* 1029-1037.

[254] Gupta, V.K. (2006). Amphetamine, migraine, and brain noradrenergic activation: contradictions in headache research. *Headache, 46,* 180-181.

[255] Cregler, L.L. and Mark, H. (1986). Medical complications of cocaine abuse. *NEJM, 315,* 1495-1500.

[256] Brower, K.J. (1988). Self-medication of migraine headaches with freebase cocaine. *J. Substance Abuse Treat, 3,* 23-26.

[257] Lance, J.W. and Curran, D.A. (1964). Treatment of chronic tension headache. *Lancet, i,* 1236-1239.

[258] Lynch, M.E. Antidepressants as analgesics: a review of randomized controlled trials. *J. Psychiatry Neurosci, 26,* 30-36.

[259] Moffett, A.M., Swash, M. and Scott, D.E. (1972). Effect of tyramine on migraine: a double-blind study. *J. Neurol. Neurosurg. Psychiatry, 35,* 496-499.

[260] Moffett, A.M., Swash, M. and Scott, D.E. (1974). Effect of chocolate on migraine: a double-blind study. *J. Neurol. Neurosurg. Psychiatry, 37,* 445-448.

[261] Wolf, M.E. and Mosnaim, A.D. (1983). Phenylethylamine in neuropsychiatric disorders. *Gen. Pharmacol, 14,* 385-390.

[262] Gupta VK. (2006). Stress-induced hypotension: Pearls and pitfalls in the theorizing process. *J. Neurol. Neurosurg. Psychiatry.* (1 March 2006). Available at: http://jnnp.bmjjournals.com/cgi/eletters/77/4/552#865

[263] Fanciullacci, M. (1979). Iris adrenergic impairment in idiopathic headache. *Headache, 19,* 8-13.

[264] Herman, P. (1983). The pupil and headaches. *Headache, 23,* 102-105.

[265] Drummond, P.D. (1991). Cervical sympathetic deficit in unilateral migraine headache. *Headache, 31,* 669-672.

[266] Drummond, P.D. (1990). Disturbances in ocular sympathetic function and facial blood flow in unilateral migraine headache. *J. Neurol. Neurosurg. Psychiatry, 53,* 121-125.

[267] Drummond, P.D. (1987). Pupil diameter in migraine and tension headache. *J. Neurol. Neurosurg. Psychiatry, 50,* 228-230.

[268] Walsh, J.P. and O'Doherty D.S. (1960). A possible explanation of the mechanism of ophthalmoplegic migraine. *Neurology, 10,* 1079-1084.

[269] Drummond, P.D. (1991). Reply: Pupillary disturbances in migraine: what is the relation to autonomic dysfunction? *J. Neurol. Neurosurg. Psychiatry, 54,* 848.

[270] Akova-Oztürk, E., Husstedt, I.W., Ringelstein, E.B. and Evers, S. (2004). Carotid artery dissection in ergotamine abuse. *Headache, 44,* 930-932.

[271] Silverman, I,E. and Wityk, R.J. (1998). Transient migraine-like symptoms with internal carotid artery dissection. *Clin. Neurol. Neurosurg, 100,* 116-120.

[272] Duyff, R.F., Snijders, C.J. and Vanneste, J.A. (1997). Spontaneous bilateral internal carotid artery dissection and migraine: a potential diagnostic delay. *Headache, 37,* 109-112.

[273] Ramadan, N.M., Tietjen, G.E., Levine, S.R. and Welch, K.M.A. (1991). Scintillating scotomata associated with internal carotid artery dissection: report of three cases. *Neurology, 41,* 1084-1087.

[274] Drummond, P.D. (1988). Dysfunction of the sympathetic nervous system in cluster headache. *Cephalalgia, 8,* 181-186.

[275] Takeshima, T., Takao, Y. and Takahashi, K. (1987). Pupillary sympathetic hypofunction and asymmetry in muscle contraction headache and migraine. *Cephalalgia, 7,* 257-262.

[276] Shimomura, T. and Takahashi, K. (1986). Pupillary functional asymmetry in patients with muscle contraction headache. *Cephalalgia, 6,* 141-145.

[277] Herman, P. (1987). Migraine, large pupils, mitral valve prolapse and emotional disturbances: an autonomic disorder. *Headache, 27,* 340-344.

[278] Bussone, G., La Mantia, L., Grazzi, L., Lamperti, E. and Boiardi, A. (1987). Internal ophthalmoplegia in complicated migraine: a case report. *Headache, 27,* 489-490.

[279] Massey, E.W. (1981). Pupillary dysautonomia and migraine: is Adie's pupil caused by migraine? *Headache, 21,* 143-146.

[280] Spierings, E.L.H. and Zieper, I. (1977). The case of the dilated pupil. *Headache, 17,* 141-144.

[281] Hallet, M. and Cogan, D.G. (1970). Episodic unilateral mydriasis in otherwise normal patients. *Arch. Ophthal, 84,* 130-136.

[282] Walsh, F.B. and Hoyt, W.F. (1969). *Clinical Neuro-ophthalmology.* (3rd ed.). Baltimore: Williams and Wilkins Co., 523-524.

[283] Alpers, B.J. and Yaskin, H.E. (1951). Pathogenesis of ophthalmoplegic migraine. *Arch. Ophthal, 45,* 555-558.

[284] Donahue, H.C. (1950). Migraine and its ocular manifestations. *Arch. Ophthal, 43,* 96-144.

[285] Rothman, M. (1903). Ueber contraction des sphincter irises lichtstarrer pupillen bei accommodation-und convergenz reaction. *Neurol. Zentralbl, 22,* 242-248.

[286] Sugiyama, N., Hamano, S., Tanaka, M., Mochizuki, M. and Nara, T. (2002). MRI findings and effectiveness of cyproheptadine in two patients with ophthalmoplegic migraine. *No To Hattatsu, 34,* 533-537.

[287] Lee, T.G., Choi, W.S. and Chung, K.C. (2002). Ophthalmoplegic migraine with reversible enhancement of intraparenchymal abducens nerve on MRI. *Headache, 42,* 140-141.

[288] O'Hara, M.A., Anderson, R.T. and Brown, D. (2001). Magnetic resonance imaging in ophthalmoplegic migraine of children. *J. AAPOS, 5,* 307-310.

[289] Tsuru, T., Nozaki, Y., Kobayashi, Y., Mizuguchi, M. and Momoi, M.Y. (1999). A case of ophthalmoplegic migraine: swelling and Gd-DTPA enhancement of the oculomotor nerve on MRI. *No To Hattatsu, 31,* 54-58.

[290] Mark, A.S., Casselman, J., Brown, D., Sanchez, J., Kolsky, M., Larsen, T.C. III, Lavin, P. and Ferraraccio, B. (1998). Ophthalmoplegic migraine: reversible enhancement and thickening of the cisternal segment of the oculomotor nerve on contrast-enhanced MR images. *Am. J. Neuroradiol, 19,* 1887-1891.

[291] Gupta, V.K. (2005). Recurrent facial palsy in migraine: mechanistic considerations. *Headache, 45,* 258-259.

[292] Vijayan, N. (1980). Ophthalmoplegic migraine: ischaemic or compressive neuropathy? *Headache, 20,* 300-304.

[293] Jacome, D.E. (2002). Status migrainosus and Adie's syndrome. *Headache, 42,* 793-795.

[294] Purvin, V.A. (1995). Adie's tonic pupil secondary to migraine. *J. Neuroophthalmol, 15,* 43-44.

[295] Bannister, R. (1988). Autonomic failure. (2nd ed.) New York: Oxford University Press, pp 3-4.

[296] Gupta, V.K. (1996). Painless Horner's syndrome in cluster headache. *J. Neurol Neurosur.g Psychiatry*, 60, 462-463.

[297] Gupta, V.K. (1991). Pupillary disturbances in migraine: what is the relation to autonomic dysfunction? *J. Neurol. Neurosurg. Psychiatry, 54,* 847-848.

[298] Duke-Elder, S. (1971). System of Ophthalmology. *Neuro-ophthalmology.* Vol X11. London: Henry Kimpton, 632-635, 653, 676-681.

[299] Riley, F.C. and Moyer, N.J. (1971). Oculosympathetic paresis associated with cluster headaches. *Am. J. Ophthalmol, 72,* 763-768.

[300] Lance, J.W., Lambert, G.A., Goadsby, P.J. and Duckworth, J.W. (1983). Brainstem influences on the cerebral circulation: experimental data from cat and monkey of relevance to the mechanism of migraine. *Headache, 23,* 258-265.

[301] Fanciullacci, M., Fusco, B.M., Alessandri, M., Campagnolo, V. and Sicuteri, F. (1989). Unilateral impairment of pupillary response to trigeminal nerve stimulation in cluster headache. *Pain, 36,* 185-191.

[302] Gupta, V.K. (2006). Visual field dysfunction and migraine: basic pathophysiological, pharmacological and clinical considerations. *Ophthal. Physiol. Opt, 26,* 217-218.

[303] Gupta, V.K. (1992). Disfunzioni visive nell'emicrania: possibile influenza della pressione intraoculare (Visual function impairment in migraine: possible role of intraocular pressure disturbance). *Confinia Cephalalgica, 1,* 259-261.

[304] Mylecharane, E.J. (1991). 5-HT$_2$ receptor antagonists and migraine therapy. *J. Neurol,* 238 Suppl 1, S45-S52.

[305] Shur, E., Checkley, S. and Delgado, I. (1983). Failure of mianserin to affect autonomic function in the pupils of depressed patients. *Acta Psychiatr. Scand, 67,* 50-55.

[306] Kopera, H. (1978). Anticholinergic and blood pressure effects of mianserin, amitriptyline and placebo. *Brit. J. Clin. Pharmacol, 5,* 29S-34S.

[307] Reynolds, J.E.F. Martindale. The Extra Pharmacopoeia. (29th Ed). London: The Pharmaceutical Press, 1989, pp 372-375.

[308] Górska, D. and Andrzejczak, D. (2003). Influence of mianserin on the activity of some hypotensive drugs in spontaneously hypertensive rats. *Pol. J. Pharmacol, 55,* 409- 417.

[309] Millson, D.S., Haworth, S.J., Rushton, A., Wilkinson, D., Hobson, S. and Harry, J. (1991). The effects of a 5-HT$_2$ receptors antagonist (ICI 169,369) on changes in waking EEG, pupillary responses and state of arousal in human volunteers. *Br. J. Clin. Pharmacol, 32,* 444-454.

[310] Millson, D.S., Jessup, C.L., Swaisland, A., Haworth, S., Rushton, A. and Harry, J.D. (1992). The effects of a selective 5-HT$_2$ receptor antagonist (ICI 170,809) on platelet aggregation and pupillary responses in healthy volunteers. *Br. J. Clin.* Pharmacol, 33, 281-288.

[311] Fanciullacci, M., Sicuteri, R., Alessandri, M. and Geppetti, P. (1995). Buspirone, but not sumatriptan, induces miosis in humans: relevance for a serotonergic pupil control. *Clin. Pharmacol. Ther, 57,* 349-355.

[312] Bodner, R.A., Lynch, T., Lewis, L. and Kahn, D. (1995). Serotonin syndrome. *Neurology,* 45, 219-223.

[313] McDaniel, W.W. (2001). Serotonin syndrome: early management with cyproheptadine. *Ann. Pharmacother, 35,* 1672-1673.

[314] Osborne, N.N. (1994). Serotonin and melatonin in the iris/ciliary processes and their involvement in intraocular pressure. *Acta Neurobiol. Exp, 54(suppl),* 57-64.

[315] Kramer, R., Rubicek, M. and Turner, P. (1973). The role of norfenfluramine in fenfluramine-induced mydriasis. *J. Pharm. Pharmacol, 25,* 575-576.

[316] Brion, N., Culig., J. and Turner, P. (1985). Indalpine effects on pupil diameter. *Therapie,* 40, 9-11.

[317] Rosenberg, M.L. and Jabbari, B. (1991). Miosis and internal ophthalmoplegia as a manifestation of partial seizures. *Neurology, 41,* 737-739.

[318] Gastaut, H., Broughton, R., Tassinari, C.A. and Roger, J. (1975). Generalized convulsive and non-convulsive seizures. In: *Handbook of clinical epilepsy.* Amsterdam: North Holland, 15, 107-144.

[319] Lesser, R. Psychogenic seizures. (1985). In: Pedley, T, Meldrum BS, eds. *Recent advances in epilepsy.* Edinburg: Churchill Livingstone, 2, 273-296.

[320] Almegård, B. and Bill, A. (1993). C-terminal calcitonin gene-related peptide fragments and vasopressin but not somatostatin-28 induce miosis in monkeys. *Eur. J. Pharmacol,* 250, 31-35.

[321] Bremner, F. and Smith, S. (2006). Pupil findings in a consecutive series of 150 cases of generalised autonomic neuropathy. *J. Neurol. Neurosurg. Psychiatry.* published online 5 Jun 2006; doi:10.1136/jnnp.2006.092833

[322] Gupta VK. (2006). Pupillary aberrations and ANS function: challenges to traditional thinking. *J. Neurol. Neurosurg. Psychiatry.* (12 June 2006). Available at: http://jnnp.bmjjournals.com/cgi/eletters/jnnp.2006.092833v1

[323] Scinto, L.F.M., Daffner, K.R., Dressler, D., Ransil, B.I., Rentz, D., Weintraub, S., Mesulam, M. and Potter, H. (1994). A potential noninvasive neurobiological test for Alzheimer's disease. *Science, 266,* 1051-1054.

[324] Litvan, I. and FitzGibbon, E.J. (1996). Can tropicamide eye drop response differentiate patients with progressive supranuclear palsy and Alzheimer's disease from healthy control subjects? *Neurology, 47,* 1324-1326.

[325] Okada, F., Shintomi, Y., Noguchi, K., Ito, Y. and Ito, N. (1989). Two cases of Hashimoto's thyroiditis with pupillary disturbances. *Eur. Neurol, 29,* 174-176.

[326] Miralles, R., Espadaler, J.M., Navarro, X. and Rubiés-Prat, J. (1995). Autonomic neuropathy in chronic alcoholism: evaluation of cardiovascular, pupillary and sympathetic skin responses. *Eur. Neurol, 35,* 287-292.

[327] Havelius, U., Heuck, M., Milos, P. and Hindfelt, B. (1997). The enhanced ciliospinal reflex in asymptomatic patients with cluster headache is due to preganglionic sympathetic mechanisms. *Headache, 37,* 496-498.

[328] Havelius, U., Milos, P. and Hindfelt, B. (1996). Cluster headache in two sisters. Pupillary response to phenylephrine and tyramine. *Headache, 36,* 448-451.

[329] Horrobin, D.F. (1973). Prevention of migraine by reducing prolactin levels? *Lancet, i,* 777.

[330] Hering, R., Gilad, I., Laron, Z. and Kuritzky, A. (1992). Effect of sodium valproate on the secretion of prolactin, cortisol and growth hormone in migraine patients. *Cephalalgia, 12,* 257-258.

[331] Ludin, H.P. Flunarizine and propranolol in the treatment of migraine. (1989). *Headache, 29,* 219-224.

[332] Bonuccelli, U., Piccini, P., Paoletti, A.M., Nuti, A., Colzi, A., Melis, G.B. and Muratorio, A. (1988). Flunarizine increases PRL secretion in normal and in migraineous women. *J. Neural. Transm, 74,* 43-53.

[333] Drago, F., Cavallaro, N., Dal Bello, A., Cavaliere, S., Spampinato, D. and Gorgone, G. (1987). Hyperprolactinemia increases intraocular pressure in humans. *Metab. Pediatr. Syst. Opthalmol, 10,* 76-77.

[334] McCallum, R.W., Sowers, J.R., Hershman, J.M. and Sturdevant, R.A. (1976). Metoclopramide stimulates prolactin secretion in man. *J. Clin. Endo. Metab, 42,* 1148-1152.

[335] Papakostas, Y., Daras, M., Markianos, M. and Stefanis, C. (1987). Increased prolactin response to thyrotropin releasing hormone during migraine attacks. *J. Neurol. Neurosurg. Psychiatry, 50,* 927-928.

[336] Peres, M.F.P., Sanchez del Rio, M., Seabra, M.L.V., Tufik, S., Abucham, J., Cipolla-Neto, J., Silberstein, S.D. and Zukerman, E. (2001). Hypothalamic involvement in chronic migraine. *J. Neurol. Neurosurg. Psychiatry, 71,* 747-751.

[337] Ader, R., Cohen, N. and Felten, D. (1995). Psychoneuroimmunology: interactions between the nervous system and the immune system. *Lancet, 345,* 99-103.

[338] Samples, J.R., Krause, G. and Lewy, A.J. (1988). Effect of melatonin on intraocular pressure. *Cur. Eye Res, 7,* 649-653.

[339] Lewy, A.J., Wehr, T.A., Goodwin, F.K., Newsome, D.A. and Markey, S.P. (1980). Light suppresses melatonin secretion in humans. *Science, 210,* 1267-1269.

[340] Claustrat, B., Loisy, C., Brun, J., Beorchia, S., Arnaud, J.L. and Chazot, G. (1989). Nocturnal plasma melatonin levels in migraine: A preliminary report. *Headache, 29,* 241-244.

[341] Lerner, A.B. and Case, J.D. (1960). Melatonin. *Fed. Proc, 19,* 590-592.

[342] Zhdanova, I.V., Wurtman, R.J., Lynch, H.J., Ives, J.R., Dollins, A.B., Morabito, C., Matheson, J.K. and Schomer, D.L. (1995). Sleep-inducing effects of low doses of melatonin ingested in the evening. *Clin. Pharmacol. Ther, 57,* 552-558.

[343] Peres, M. F.P., Zukerman, E., Tanuri, F. C., Moreira, F. R. and Cipolla-Neto, J. (2004). Melatonin, 3 mg, is effective for migraine prevention. *Neurology, 63,* 757.

[344] Juszczak, M., Bojanowska, E. and Ryszard Dabrowski, R. (2000). Melatonin and the synthesis of vasopressin in pinealectomized male rats. *PSEBM, 225, 207-210.*

[345] Juszczak, M., Debeljuk, L., Stempniak, B., Steger, R.W., Fadden, C. and Bartke, A. (1997). Neurohypophyseal vasopressin in the Syrian hamster: response to short photoperiod, pinealectomy, melatonin treatment, or osmotic stimulation. *Brain Res. Bull, 42,* 221-225.

[346] Watanabe, K., Yamaoka, S. and Vanecek, J. (1998). Melatonin inhibits spontaneous and VIP-induced vasopressin release from suprachiasmatic neurons. *Brain Res, 801,* 216-219.

[347] Juszczak, M, Appenrodt, E., Guzek, J.W. and Schwarzberg, H. (1999). Effects of oxytocin and vasopressin on retrieval of passive avoidance response in melatonin-treated and/or pinealectomized male rats. *Neuroendo Lett, 20,* 77-81.

[348] Girardin Jean-Louis, G., Daniel F Kripke, D.F., Elliott, J.A., Zizi, F., Wolintz, A.H. and Lazzaro, D.R. (2005). Daily illumination exposure and melatonin: influence of ophthalmic dysfunction and sleep duration. *J Circadian Rhythms, 3,* 13.

[349] Giffin, N.J., Ruggiero, L., Lipton,, R.B., Silberstein, S.D., Tvedskov, J.F., Olesen, J., Altman, J., Goadsby, P.J. and Macrae, A. (2003). Premonitory symptoms in migraine. An electronic diary study. *Neurology, 60,* 935-940.

[350] Coppola, G., Vandenheede, M., Di Clemente, L., Ambrosini, A., Fumal, A., De Pasqua, V. and Schoenen, J. (2005). Somatosensory evoked high-frequency oscillations reflecting thalamo-cortical activity are decreased in migraine patients between attacks. *Brain, 128,* 98-103.

[351] Schoenen, J., Ambrosini, A., Sàndor, P.S. and Maertens de Noordhout, A. (2003). Evoked potentials and transcranial magnetic stimulation in migraine: published data and viewpoint on their pathophysiologic significance. *Clin. Neurophysiol, 114,* 955-972.

[352] Ozkul, Y. and Uckardes, A. (2002). Median nerve somatosensory evoked potentials in migraine. *Eur. J. Neurol, 9,* 227-232.

[353] Ambrosini, A., Rossi, P., De Pasqua, V., Pierelli, F. and Schoenen, J. (2003). Lack of habituation causes high intensity dependence of auditory evoked cortical potentials in migraine. *Brain, 2003,* 2009-2015.

[354] Gawel, M., Connolly, J.F. and Clifford Rose, F.C. (1983). Migraine patients exhibit abnormalities in the visual evoked potential. *Headache, 23,* 49-52.

[355] Drake, M.E., Pakalnis, A., Hietter, S.A. and Padamadan, H. (1990). Visual and auditory evoked potentials in migraine. *Electromyog Clin. Neurophysiol, 30,* 77-81.

[356] Gupta, V.K. (1993). Visual function impairment in migraine: cerebral versus retinal defect. *Cephalalgia, 13,* 431-432.

[357] Maertens de Noordhout, A., Timsit-Berthier, M. and Schoenen, J. (1985). Contingent negative variation (CNV) in migraineurs before and during prophylactic treatment with β-blockers. *Cephalalgia, 5,* 34-35.

[358] Schoenen, J., Timsit-Berthier, M. and Timsit, M. (1985). Correlations between contingent negative variation and plasma levels of catecholamines in headache patients. *Cephalalgia, 5 (suppl 3),* 480.

[359] Böcker, K.B.E., Timsit-Berthier, M., Schoenen, J. and Brunia, C.H.M. (1990). Contingent negative variation in migraine. *Headache, 30,* 604-609.

[360] Mosnaim, A.D., Diamond, S., Wolf, M.E., Puente, J. and Freitag, F.G. (1989). Endogenous opioid-like peptides in headache. An overview. *Headache, 29,* 368-372.

[361] Kobari, M., Meyer, J.S., Ichijo, M., Imai, A. and Oravez, W.T. (1989). Hyperperfusion of cerebral cortex, thalamus and basal ganglia during spontaneously occurring migraine headaches. *Headache, 29,* 282-289.

[362] Passchier, J. (1994). A critical note on psychophysiological stress research into migraine patients. *Headache, 14,* 194-198.

[363] Schwarzer, R. (1998). Stress and coping from a social cognitive perspective. *Ann. N. Y. Acad. Sci, 851,* 531-537.

[364] Steiner, T.J. (2004). Lifting the burden: the global campaign against headache. *Lancet Neurology, 3,* 204-205.

[365] Lance, J.W. (1996). Migraine: then and now. *MJA, 164,* 519-520.

[366] Schrader, H., Stovner, L.J., Helde, G., Sand, T. and Bovim, G. (2001). Prophylactic treatment of migraine with angiotensin converting enzyme inhibitor (lisinopril): randomised, placebo controlled, crossover study. *BMJ, 322,* 19-22.

[367] Bigal, M.E., Rapoport, A.M., Sheftell, F.D. and Tepper, S.J. (2002). New migraine preventative options: an update with pathophysiological considerations. *Rev. Hosp. Clin. Fac. Med. Sao. Paulo, 57,* 293-298.

[368] Sakaguchi, K., Chai, S.Y., Jackson, B., Johnston, C.I. and Mendelsohn, F.A. (1987). Blockade of angiotensin converting enzyme in circumventricular organs of the brain after oral lisinopril administration demonstrated by quantitative in vitro Autoradiography. *Clin. Exp. Pharmacol. Physiol, 14,* 155-158

[369] Tronvik, E., Stovner, L.J., Helde, G., Sand, T. and Bovim, G. (2003). Prophylactic treatment of migraine with an angiotensin II receptor blocker: a randomized controlled trial. *JAMA, 289,* 65-69.

[370] Tocco, D.J., Clineschmidt, B.V., Duncan, A.E.W., DeLuna, F.A. and Baer, J.E. (1980). Uptake of beta-adrenergic blocking agents propranolol and timolol by rodent brain: relationship to central pharmacological actions. *J. Cardiovasc. Pharmacol, 2,* 133-143.

[371] Chi, O.Z., Wang, G., Chang, Q. and Weiss, H.R. (1998). Effects of isoproterenol on blood-brain barrier permeability in rats. *Neurol. Res, 20,* 259-264.

[372] Schoenen, J., Jacquy, J. and Lenaerts M. (1998). Effectiveness of high-dose riboflavin in migraine prophylaxis. A randomized controlled trial. *Neurology, 50,* 466-470.

[373] Spector, R. (1980). Riboflavin homeostasis in the central nervous system. *J. Neurochem, 35,* 202-209.

[374] van Bree, J.B.M.M., De Boer, A.G., Verhoef, J.C., Danhof, M and Breimer, D.D. (1989). Transport of vasopressin fragments across the blood-brain barrier: *in vitro* studies using monolayer cultures of bovine brain endothelial cells. *J. Pharm. Exp. Ther, 249,* 901-905.

[375] Nagao, S. (1988). Vasopressin and blood-brain barrier. *No To Shinkei, 50,* 809-815. (Abstract—Article in Japanese).

[376] Adelman, L.C., Adelman, J.U., Seggern, V. (R) and Mannix, L.X. (2000). Venlafaxine extended release (XR) for the prophylaxis of migraine and tension-type headache: A retrospective study in a clinical setting. *Headache, 40,* 572-580.

[377] Merikangas, K.R. and Merikangas, J.R. (1995). Combination monoamine oxidase inhibitor and beta-blocker treatment of migraine, with anxiety and depression. *Biol. Psychiatry, 38,* 603-610.

[378] Mathew, N.T. (1981). Prophylaxis of migraine and mixed headache. A randomized controlled study. *Headache, 21,* 105-109.

[379] Nag, S. (1991). Protective effect of flunarizine on blood-brain barrier permeability alterations in acutely hypertensive rats. *Stroke, 22,* 1265-1269.

[380] Tassorelli, C., Blandini, F., Costa, A., Preza, E. and Nappi, G. (2002). Nitroglycerin-induced activation of monoaminergic transmission in the rat. *Cephalalgia, 22,* 226- 232.

[381] Mayhan, W.G. (2000). Nitric oxide donor-induced increase in permeability of the blood-brain barrier. *Brain Res, 866,* 101-108.

[382] Boje, K.M. (1996). Inhibition of nitric oxide synthase attenuates blood-brain barrier disruption during experimental meningitis. *Brain Res, 720,* 75-83.

[383] Thiel, V.E. and Audus, K.L. (2001). Nitric oxide and blood-brain barrier integrity. *Antioxidants and Redox Signaling, 3,* 273-278.

[384] Bigal, M.E. and Krymchantowski, A.V. (2006). Emerging drugs for migraine prophylaxis and treatment. *MedGenMed, 8,* 31. Available at: http://www.medscape.com/viewarticle/528452 (Accessed September 29, 2006).

[385] Gilron, I. (2006). The role of anticonvulsant drugs in postoperative pain management: a bench-to-bedside perspective. *Can. J. Anesth, 53,* 562-571.

[386] Aley, K.O. and Kulkarni, S.K. (1989). GABAergic agents-induced antinociceptive effect in mice. *Meth. Find Exp. Clin. Pharmacol, 11,* 597-601.

[387] Brandes, J.L. (2006). The influence of estrogen on migraine. A systematic review. *JAMA, 295,* 1824-1830.

[388] Bannwarth, B., Demotes-Mainard, F., Schaeverbeke, T., Labat, L. and Dehais, J. (1995). Central analgesic effects of aspirin-like drugs. *Fundam. Clin. Pharmacol, 9,* 1-7.

[389] Page, I.H. (1954). Serotonin (5-hydroxytryptamine). *Physiol. Rev, 34,* 563-588.

[390] Humphrey, P.P.A. (1991). 5-hydroxytryptamine and the pathophysiology of migraine. *J. Neurol, 238,* S38-S44.

[391] Sicuteri, F., Testi, A. and Anselmi, B. (1961). Biochemical investigations in headache: increase in the hydroxyindoleacetic acid excretion during migraine attacks. *Int. Arch. Allergy, 19,* 55-58.

[392] Curran, D.A., Hinterberger, H. and Lance, J.W. (1965). Total plasma serotonin, 5-hydroxyindoleacetic acid, and *p*-hydroxy-*m*-metoxymandelic acid excretion in normal and migrainous subjects. *Brain, 88,* 997-1010.

[393] Arulmani, U., Gupta, S., VanDenBrink, A.M., Centurión, D., Villalón, C.M. and Saxena, P.R. (2006). Experimental migraine models and their relevance in migraine therapy. *Cephalalgia, 26,* 642-659.

[394] Lance, J.W. (1988). Fifty years of migraine research. *Aust. NZ J. Med, 18,* 311-317.

[395] Malmgren, R. and Hasselmark, L. (1988). The platelet and the neuron: two cells in focus in migraine. *Cephalalgia, 8,* 7-24.

[396] Da Prada, M., Cesura, A.M., Launay, J.M. and Richards, J.G. (1988). Platelets as a model for neurons? *Experientia, 44,* 115-127.

[397] Joseph, R., Welch, K.M.A. and D'Andrea, G. (1989). Serotonergic hypofunction in migraine: a synthesis of evidence based on platelet dense body dysfunction. *Cephalalgia, 9,* 293-299.

[398] Panconesi, A. (1995). 5-hydroxytryptamine parameters in the periphery: how useful are they in the study of headaches? *J. Serotonin Res, 2,* 117-137.

[399] Ferrari, M.D., Odink, J., Tapparelli, C., Van Kempen, G.M.J., Pennings, E.J.M. and Bruyn, G.W. (1989). Serotonin metabolism in migraine. *Neurology, 39,* 1239-1242.

[400] Ranson, R., Igarashi, H., MacGregor, E.A. and Wilkinson, M. (1991). The similarities and differences of migraine with aura and migraine without aura: a preliminary study. *Cephalalgia, 11,* 189-192.

[401] Rasmussen, B.K., Jensen, R. and Olesen, J. (1991). A population-based analysis of the diagnostic criteria of the International Headache Society. *Cephalalgia, 11,* 129-134.

[402] Lance, J.W. (1990). A concept of migraine and the search for the ideal headache drug. *Headache, 30,* 17-23.

[403] Ferrari, M.D. and Saxena, P.R. (1993). On serotonin and migraine: a clinical and pharmacological review. *Cephalalgia, 13,* 151-165.

[404] Kimball, R.W., Friedman, A.P. and Vallejo, E. (1960). Effect of serotonin in migraine patients. *Neurology, 10,* 107-111.

[405] Hopf, H.C., Johnson, E.A. and Gutmann, L. (1992). Protective effect of serotonin on migraine attacks. *Neurology, 42,* 1419.

[406] Busse, R., Mulsch, A., Fleming, I. and Hecker, M. (1993). Mechanisms of nitric oxide release from the vascular endothelium. *Circulation, 87,* (Suppl V), 18-25.

[407] Stroes, E.S.G., Koomans, H.A., de Bruin, T.W.A. and Rabelink, T.J. (1995). Vascular function in the forearm of hypercholesterolaemic patients off and on lipid-lowering medication. *Lancet, 346,* 467-471.

[408] Gupta, V.K. (2005). Glyceryl trinitrate and migraine: nitric oxide donor precipitating and aborting migrainous aura. *J Neurol Neurosurg Psychiatry* (22 October 2005). Available at: http://www.jnnp.com/cgi/eletters /76/8/1158#708 (Accessed 27 September, 2006).

[409] Ulmer, H.J., de Lima, V.M. and Hanke, W. (1995). Effects of nitric oxide on the retinal spreading depression. *Brain Res, 691,* 239-242.

[410] Grotemeyer, K-H., Scharafinski, H-W., Schlake, H-P., and Husstedt, I.W. (1990). Acetylsalicylic acid vs. metoprolol in migraine prophylaxis -- a double-blind cross-over study. *Headache, 30,* 639-641.

[411] Steiner, T.J., Joseph, R. and Clifford Rose, F. (1985). Migraine is not a platelet disorder. *Headache, 25,* 434-440.

[412] Laustiola, K,, Seppala, B., Nikkari, T. and Vapataalo, H. (1984). Exercise-induced increase in plasma arachidonic acid and thromboxan B_2 in healthy

men: effect of beta-adrenergic blockade. *J. Cardiovasc. Pharmacol, 6,* 449-454.

[413] Gawel, M., Burkitt, M. and Clifford Rose, F. (1979). The platelet release reaction during migraine attacks. *Headache, 19,* 323-327.

[414] Hioki, H., Aoki, N., Kawano, K., Homori, M., Hasumura, Y., Yasumura, T., Maki, A., Yoshino, H., Yanagisawa, A. and Ishikawa, K. (2001). Acute effects of cigarette smoking on platelet-dependent thrombin generation. *Eur. Heart J, 22,* 56-61.

[415] Scher, A.I., Terwindt, G.M., Picavet H.S.J., Verschuren W.M.M., Ferrari, M.D. and Launer, L.J. (2005). Cardiovascular risk factors and migraine. The GEM population- based study. Neurology, 64, 614-620.

[416] Volans, G.N. and Castleden, C.M. (1976). The relationship between smoking and migraine. *Postgrad. Med. J, 52,* 80-82.

[417] Markus, H.S. and Hopkinson, N. (1992). Migraine and headache in systemic lupus erythematosus and their relationship with antibodies against phospholipids. *J. Neurol, 239,* 39-42.

[418] Gupta, V.K. (2004). Platelet-leukocyte adhesion, migraine, and stroke: a bioclinical perspective. *J. Neurol. Neurosurg. Psychiatry.* [12 July 2004]. Available at: http://jnnp.bmjjournals.com/cgi/eletters/75/7/984#197 (Accessed 25 September, 2006).

[419] Appenzeller, O. (1991). Pathogenesis of migraine. *Med. Clin. North Am, 75,* 763-789.

[420] Silberstein, S.D. and Merriam, G.R. (1991). Estrogens, progestins, and headache. *Neurology, 41,* 786-93.

[421] Altura, B.M. and Altura, B.T. (1977). Some physiological factors in vascular reactivity. V. Influences of sex hormones, oral contraceptives and pregnancy on vascular muscle and its reactivity. In: Carrier O and Shibata S. (eds) *Factors influencing vascular reactivity.* Tokyo: Igaku-Shoin Ltd.

[422] Jennings, L.K., White, M.M., Sauer, C.M., Mauer, A.M. and Robertson, J.T. (1993). Cocaine-induced platelet defects. *Stroke, 24,* 1352-1359.

[423] Ziegler, D.K. (1990). Headache. Public health problem. *Neurol. Clin, 8,* 781-91.

[424] Broderick, J.P. and Swanson, J.W. (1987). Migraine-related strokes. Clinical profile and prognosis in 20 patients. *Arch. Neurol, 44,* 868-871.

[425] Gupta, V.K. (2004). On the non-specific link between migraine and depression. *J. Neurol. Neurosurg. Psychiatry.* (23 January 2004). Available at: http://jnnp. bmjjournals.com/ cgi/eletters/74/11/1587#91

[426] Wessely S. Britain on the couch: treating a low serotonin society. Br Med J 1998;316:83.

[427] Aghajanian, G.K. and Wang, R.Y. (1978). Physiology and pharmacology of central serotoninergic neurons. In *Psychopharmacology: A Generation of Progress*, edited by M.A. Lipton, A. DiMascio, and K.F.Killiam. New York: Raven Press.

[428] Panconesi, A. and Sicuteri, R. (1997). Headache induced by serotonergic agonists—a key to the interpretation of migraine pathogenesis? *Cephalalgia, 17*, 3-14.

[429] Peroutka, S.J. (1988). Antimigraine drug interactions with serotonin receptor subtypes in human brain. *Ann. Neurol, 23*, 500-504.

[430] Dougherty, J.A., Young, H. and Shafi, T. (2002). Serotonin syndrome induced by amitriptyline, meperidine, and venlafaxine. *Ann. Pharmacother, 36*, 1647-1648.

[431] Perry, N.K. (2000). Venlafaxine-induced serotonin syndrome with relapse following amitriptyline. *Postgrad. Med. J, 76*, 254-256.

[432] Sternbach, H. (1991). The serotonin syndrome. *Am. J. Psychiatry, 148*, 705-713.

[433] Mathew, N.T., Tietjen, G.E. and Lucker, C. (1996). Serotonin syndrome complicating migraine pharmacotherapy. *Cephalalgia, 16*, 323-327.

[434] Gupta, V.K. (2006). Amitriptyline versus cyproheptadine: opposite influences on brain 5-HT function. *Headache*, (In press).

[435] Davies, P.T.G. and Steiner, T.J. (1990). Serotonin S2 receptors and migraine: a study with the selective antagonist ICI 169,369. *Headache, 30*, 340-343.

[436] Fozard, J.R. (1990). 5-HT in migraine: evidence from 5-HT receptor antagonists for a neuronal aetiology. In: Sandler, M. and Collins, G.M. (eds) *Migraine: a spectrum of ideas.* Oxford University Press, Oxford, 128-146.

[437] Lynch, M.E. (2001). Antidepressants as analgesics: a review of randomized controlled trials. *J. Psychiatry Neurosci, 26*, 30-36.

[438] Baumeister, A.A., Hawkins, M.F. and Uzelac, S.M. (2003). The myth of reserpine induced depression: role in the historical development of the monoamine hypothesis. *J. Hist. Neurosci, 12*, 207-220.

[439] Hyman, E.S. (1979). The drinking water-cancer-carbon filtration problem. *J. La. State Med Soc., 131*, 11-32.

[440] Facchinetti, F., Neril, I., Martignoni, E., Fioroni, L., Nappi, G. and Genazzani, A.R. (1993) The association of menstrual migraine with the premenstrual syndrome. *Cephalalgia, 13*, 422-425.

[441] Gupta, V.K. (2004). Menstrual migraine is not pathogenetically related to premenstrual syndrome. *Cephalalgia, 14*, 411-414.

[442] Facchinetti, F., Nappi, G., Petralgia, F., Volpe, A. and Genazzani, A.R. (1983). Estradiol/progesterone imbalance and the premenstrual syndrome. *Lancet , ii,* 1302-3.

[443] Facchinetti, F., Martignoni, E., Sola, D., Petralgia, F., Nappi, G. and Genazzani, A.R. (1988). Transient failure of central opioid tonus and premenstrual symptoms. *J Reprod Med, 33,* 633-638.

[444] Facchinetti, F., Martignoni, E., Fioroni, L., Sances, G. and Genazzani, A.R (1990). Opioid control of the hypothalamo-pituitary-adrenal axis cyclically fails in menstrual migraine. *Cephalalgia, 10,* 51-56.

[445] Facchinetti, F. (1994). The premenstrual syndrome belongs in the diagnostic criteria for menstrual migraine. *Cephalalgia, 14,* 413-414.

[446] Grossman, A. and Besser, G.M. (1982) Opiates control ACTH through a noradrenergic mechanism. *Clin Endocrinol, 17,* 287-290.

[447] Recht, L.D. and Abrams, G.M. (1986). Neuropeptides and their role in nociception and analgesia. *Neurol Clin, 4,* 833-852.

[448] Halbreich, U., Holtz, I. and Paal, L. (1988). Premenstrual changes. Impaired hormonal homeostasis. *Neurol Clin, 6,* 173-194.

[449] Smock, T. and Fields, H.L. (1980). ACTH (1-24) blocks opiate-induced analgesia in the rat. *Brain Res, 212,* 202-206.

[450] Koob, G.F. and Bloom, F.E. (1982) Behavioral effects of neuropeptides: endorphins and vasopressin. *Ann Rev Physiol, 44,* 571-582.

[451] Maier, S.F., Drugan, R.C. and Grau, J.W. (1982). Controllability, coping behavior, and stress-induced analgesia in the rat. *Pain, 12,* 47-56.

[452] Blau, J.N. (1991). The clinical diagnosis of migraine: the beginning of therapy. *J Neurol, 238,* S6-11.

[453] Spierings, E.L.H., Reinders, M.J. and Hoogduin, C.A.L. (1989). The migraine aura as a cause of avoidance behavior. *Headache, 29,* 254-255.

[454] Sommerville, B.W. (1972). The role of estradiol withdrawal in the etiology of menstrual migraine. *Neurology, 22,* 355-365.

[455] Lechat, P., Mas, J.L., Lascault, G., Loron, P., Theard, M, Klimczac, M., Drobinski, G., Thomas, D. And Grosgogeat, Y. (1988). Prevalence of patent foramen ovale in patients with stroke. *N Engl J Med, 318,* 1148- 1152.

[456] Wood, S. (2007). FDA panel says PFO occluders must prove themselves in RCTs, no matter how long it takes. Heartwire. Available at: http://www.medscape.com/viewarticle/553118

[457] Adams, H.P. (2004). Patent foramen ovale: paradoxical embolism and paradoxical data. *Mayo Clin Proc, 79,* 15-20.

[458] Gupta, V.K. (2009). Closure of PFO: science, quasi-science, or empiricism. *Cardiology, 113,* 108-110.

[459] Hellman, S. and Hellman, D.S. (1991). Of mice but not men – problems of the randomized clinical trial. *N Engl J Med, 324,* 1585-1589.

[460] Passamani, E. (1991). Clinical trials – are they ethical? *N Engl J Med, 324,* 1589-1592.

[461] Herman, J. (1994). Experiment and observation. *Lancet, 344,* 1209-1211.

[462] Gupta, V.K. (2009). ß-blockers, hypertension, and RCTs: science and sensibility. *J. Am. Coll. Cardiol.* (In press)

[463] Li ,J., Zhang, Q., Zhang, M. and Egger, M. (2007). Intravenous magnesium for acute myocardial infarction. *Cochrane Database of Systematic Reviews, Issue 2,* Art. No. CD002755. DOI:10.1002/14651858.CD002755.pub2.

[464] Serena, J., Marti-Fa`bregas, J., Santamarina, E., Rodríguez, J.J., Perez-Ayuso, M.J., Masjuan, J., Segura, T., Ga´llego, J. and Da´valos, A. on Behalf of the CODICIA (Right-to-Left Shunt in Cryptogenic Stroke) Study; for the Stroke Project of the Cerebrovascular Diseases Study Group, Spanish Society of Neurology. Recurrent Stroke and Massive Right-to-Left Shunt. (2008). Results From the Prospective Spanish Multicenter (CODICIA) Study. *Stroke, 39,* 3131-3136.

[465] Dowson, A.J., Mullen, M., Peatfield, R., Muir, K., Khan, A., Wells, C., Lipscombe, S., Rees, T., De Giovanni, J., Morrison, W., Hildick-Smith, D., Elrington, G., Hillis, W., Malik, I. and Rickards, A. (2008). Migraine Intervention with STARFlex Technology trial: a prospective, multicentre, double-blind, sham-controlled trial to evaluate the effectiveness of patent foramen ovale closure with STARFlex septal repair implant to resolve refractory migraine headache. *Circulation, 117,* 1397-1404.

[466] Mas JL, Arquizan C, Lamy C, et al. (2001). Patent Foramen Ovale and Atrial Septal Aneurysm Study Group. Recurrent cerebrovascular events associated with patent foramen ovale, atrial septal aneurysm, or both. *N Engl J Med, 345,* 1740-1746.

[467] Homma, S., Sacco, R.L., Di Tullio, M.R., Sciacca, R.R. and Mohr JP, PFO in Cryptogenic Stroke (PICSS) Investigators. (2002). Effect of medical treatment in stroke patients with patent foramen ovale: patent foramen ovale in Cryptogenic Stroke Study. *Circulation, 105,* 2625-2631.

[468] Kutty, S., Brown, K., Qureshi, A.M. and Latson, .L.A. (2009). Maximal potential patent foramen diameter does not correlate with type or frequency of neurologic event prior to closure. *Cardiology, 113,* 111-115.

[469] Di Tullio, M.R., Sacco, R.L., Sciacca, R.R., Jin, Z. and Homma S. 2007). Patent foramen ovale and the risk of ischemic stroke in a multiethnic population. *J. Am. Coll. Cardiol., 49,* 797-802.

[470] Schuchlenz HW, Weihs W, Horner S, Quehenberger F. (2000). The association between the diameter of a patent foramen ovale and the risk of embolic cerebrovascular events. *Am. J. Med., 109,* 456-462.

[471] Lamy C, Giannesini C, Zuber M, et al. (2002). Clinical and imaging findings in cryptogenic stroke patients with and without patent foramen ovale: the PFO-ASA Study. *Stroke, 33,* 706-711.

[472] Gupta, V.K. PFO and migraine: pearls and pitfalls in the theorizing process. (2005). *Heart.*

[473] http://heart.bmjjournals.com/cgi/eletters/90/11/1315#842

[474] Berdat, P.A., Chatterjee, T., Pfammatter, J.P., Windecker, S., Meier, B. and Carrel, T. (2000). Surgical management of complications after transcatheter closure of an atrial septal defect or patent foramen ovale. *J Thorac Cardiovasc Surg, 120,* 1034-1039.

[475] Stöllberger, C., Finsterer, J., Krexener, E. And Schneider, B. (2008). Stroke and peripheral embolism from an Amplatzer septal occluder 5 years after implantation. *J Neurol, 255,* 1270-1271.

[476] Holmes, D.R. Jr and Cabalka, A. (2002). Was your mother right—do we always need to close the door? *Circulation, 106,* 1034-1036.

[477] Stoeckle, J.D. (1995). Do patients want to be informed? Do they want to decide? *J Gen Intern Med, 10,* 643-644.

[478] Cassileth, B.R., Zupkis, R.V., Sutton-Smith, K. and March, V. (1980). Informed consent – why are its goals imperfectly realized. *N Engl J Med, 302,* 896-900.

[479] Vandenbroucke, J.P. (1998). Medical journals and the shaping of medical knowledge. *Lancet, 352,* 2001-2006.

[480] Davidson, R.A. (1986). Source of funding and outcome of clinical trials. (1986) *J Gen Intern Med, 1,* 155-158.

[481] Gillett, R. and Harrow, J. (1993). Is medical research well served by peer review? *Brit Med J, 306,* 1672-1675.

[482] Editorial. The side-effects of doing good. Economist (Feb 21, 2008). http://www.economist.com/world/international/displaystory.cfm?story_id=10729975

[483] Silverman, W.A. and Altman, D.G. (1996). Patients' preferences and randomized trials. *Lancet, 347,* 171-174.

[484] Martyn, C. (1996). Not quite as random as I pretended. *Lancet, 347,* 70.

[485] Kassirer, J.P. (1993). The frustrations of scientific misconduct. (1993) *N Engl J Med, 328,* 1634-1636.

[486] Silverman, W.A. and Altman, D.G. (1996). Patients' preferences and randomized trials. *Lancet, 347,* 171-174.

[487] Skrabanek, P. (1993). The Ethics and Politics of Human Experimentation. Cambridge University Press, Cambridge.

[488] Gupta, V.K. (1996). Should intellectual property be disseminated by forwarding" rejected letters without permission? *J. Med. Ethics., 22,* 243-244 (response by *Br. Med. J. 1996, 22,* 245-246; comments 360-361).

[489] Tobis, J. and Azarbal, B. (2005) Reply. *J. Am. Coll. Cardiol., 46,* 738-739.

[490] Gupta, V.K. (1995). Regional cerebral blood flow patterns in migraine: what is the contribution to insight into disease mechanisms? *Eur. J. Neurol.,* 2, 586-587 (comments 588-589).

[491] Hara, H., Virmani, R., Ladich, E., Mackey-Bojack, S., Titus, J., Reisman, M., Gray, W., Nakamura, M., Mooney, M., Poulose, A. and Schwartz, R.S. (2005). Patent foramen ovale: current pathology, pathophysiology, and clinical status. *J Am Coll Cardiol, 46,* 1768-1776.

[492] Gupta, V.K. (2005). ASD closure for migraine: is there a scientific basis? *Eur Heart J, 26,* 1446.

[493] Gupta, V., Yesilbursa, D., Huang, W.Y., et al. (2008). Patent foramen ovale in a large population of ischemic stroke patients: diagnosis, age distribution, gender, and race. *Echocardiography, 25,* 217-227.

[494] Joseph, R., Steiner, T.J., Schultz, L.U.C. and Rose, F.C. (1998). Platelet activity and selective ß- blockade in migraine prophylaxis. *Stroke, 19,* 704-708.

[495] Jayachandran, M., Sanzo, A., Owen, W. and Miller, V.M. (2005). Estrogenic regulation of tissue factor and tissue factor pathway inhibitor in platelets. *Am J Physiol [Heart Circ Physiol], 58,* H1908-H1916.

[496] Finocchi, C., Del Sette, M., Angeli, S., Rizzi, D. and Gandolfo, C. (2004).

[497] Cluster headache and right-to-left shunt on contrast transcranial Doppler. A case-control study. *Neurology, 63,* 1309-1310.

[498] Gupta, V.K. (2004). Percutaneous closure of patent foramen ovale reduces the frequency of migraine attacks. *Neurology, 63,* 1760-1761.

[499] Milhaud, D., Bogousslavsky, J., van Melle, G. and Liot, P. (2001). Ischemic stroke and active migraine. *Neurology, 57,* 1805-1811.

[500] Broderick, J.P. and Swanson, J.W. (1987). Migraine-related strokes. Clinical profile and prognosis in 20 patients. *Arch. Neurol., 44,* 868-871.

[501] J.D. Watson. The Double Helix. 1968. Signet Books, New American Library, New York.

[502] Burkitt, D. (1992). How important is IQ in research. *Br. Med. J.,* 305, 1300.

[503] Rumi. Poet and mystic. Selections from his writings. (translated by R.A. Nicholson). London: Allen and Unwin, 1950.

INDEX

D

I

N

P

O

S

T

U

V